Demos Surgical Pathology Guides

Breast Pathology

SERIES EDITOR

Saul Suster, MD
Professor and Chairman
Department of Pathology
Medical College of Wisconsin
Milwaukee, Wisconsin

TITLES

- *Head and Neck Pathology*
  Paul E. Wakely Jr.

FORTHCOMING TITLES

- *Inflammatory Skin Disorders*
  Jose A. Plaza and Victor Prieto

- *Skin Tumors*
  Jose A. Plaza and Victor Prieto

- *Pulmonary Pathology*
  R. Nagarjun Rao and Cesar A. Moran

- *Soft Tissues*
  Eduardo V. Zambrano

- *Lymph Nodes*
  Steven H. Kroft, Alexandra Harrington, and Horatiu Olteanu

- *Gastrointestinal Pathology*
  Richard A. Komorowski

Demos Surgical Pathology Guides

Breast Pathology

GIOVANNI FALCONIERI, MD
Department of Pathology
General University Hospital
Udine, Italy

JANEZ LAMOVEC, MD
Department of Pathology
Institute of Oncology
Ljubljana, Slovenia

ABIY B. AMBAYE, MD
Associate Professor of Pathology
Department of Pathology
University of Vermont
Burlington, Vermont

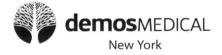
demosMEDICAL
New York

ISBN: 978-1-936287-30-7
eISBN: 978-1-617050-60-2

Acquisitions Editor: Richard Winters
Production Editor: Dana Bigelow
Compositor: S4Carlisle Publishing Services
Printer: Bradford & Bigelow

Visit our website at www.demosmedpub.com

Medicine is an ever-changing science. Research and clinical experience are continually expanding our knowledge, in particular our understanding of proper treatment and drug therapy. The authors, editors, and publisher have made every effort to ensure that all information in this book is in accordance with the state of knowledge at the time of production of the book. Nevertheless, the authors, editors, and publisher are not responsible for errors or omissions or for any consequences from application of the information in this book and make no warranty, express or implied, with respect to the contents of the publication. Every reader should examine carefully the package inserts accompanying each drug and should carefully check whether the dosage schedules mentioned therein or the contraindications stated by the manufacturer differ from the statements made in this book. Such examination is particularly important with drugs that are either rarely used or have been newly released on the market.

Library of Congress Cataloging-in-Publication Data
Falconieri, Giovanni.
Breast pathology / Giovanni Falconieri, Janez Lamovec, Abiy B. Ambaye.
      p. ; cm.
   Includes bibliographical references and index.
   ISBN-13: 978-1-936287-30-7
   ISBN-10: 1-936287-30-7
   ISBN-13: 978-1-61705-060-2 (e-ISBN)
   ISBN-10: 1-61705-060-1 (e-ISBN)
   I. Lamovec, Janez. II. Ambaye, Abiy B. III. Title.
   [DNLM: 1. Breast Neoplasms—pathology. 2. Breast Diseases—pathology. 3. Neoplasm Invasiveness.
4. Precancerous Conditions. WP 870]
   LC classification not assigned
   616.99'44907—dc23
                                                                                    2011032952

Special discounts on bulk quantities of Demos Medical Publishing books are available to corporations, professional associations, pharmaceutical companies, health care organizations, and other qualifying groups. For details, please contact:

Special Sales Department
Demos Medical Publishing
11 W. 42nd Street, 15th Floor
New York, NY 10036
Phone: 800–532–8663 or 212–683–0072
Fax: 212–941–7842
E-mail: rsantana@demosmedpub.com

Printed in the United States of America
12 13 14 15   5 4 3 2 1

Contents

Series Foreword

The field of surgical pathology has gained increasing relevance and importance over the years as pathologists have become more and more integrated into the health care team. To the need for precise histopathologic diagnoses has now been added the burden of providing our clinical colleagues with information that will allow them to assess the prognosis of the disease and predict the response to therapy. Pathologists now serve as key consultants in the patient management team and are responsible for providing critical information that will guide their therapy. With the progress gained due to the insights obtained from the application of newer diagnostic techniques, surgical pathology has become progressively more complex. As a result, diagnoses need to be more detailed and specific and the number of data elements required in the generation of a surgical pathology report have increased exponentially, making management of the information required for diagnosis cumbersome and sometimes difficult.

The past 15 years have witnessed an explosion of information in the field of pathology with a massive proliferation of specialized textbooks appearing in print. For the most part, such texts provide in-depth and detailed coverage of the various areas in surgical pathology. The purpose of this series is to bridge the gap between the major subspecialty texts and the large, double-volume general surgical pathology textbooks, by providing compact, single-volume monographs that will succinctly address the most salient and important points required for the diagnosis of the most common conditions. The series is organized following an organ-system format, with single volumes dedicated to individual organs. The volumes are divided on the basis of disease groups, including benign reactive, inflammatory, infectious or systemic conditions, benign neoplastic conditions, and malignant neoplasms. Each chapter consists of a bulleted list of the most pertinent clinical data related to the condition, followed by the most important histopathologic criteria for diagnosis, pertinent use of immunohistochemical stains and other ancillary techniques, and relevant molecular tests when available. This is followed by a section on differential diagnosis. References appear at the back of the volume. Each entity is illustrated with key, high-quality histological images that highlight the most salient and distinctive features that need to be recognized for the correct diagnosis.

These books are intended for the busy practicing pathologist, and for pathology residents and fellows in training who require an easy and simple overview of major diagnostic criteria and key points during the course of routine daily practice. The authors have been carefully chosen for their experience in the field and clarity of exposition in the various topics. It is hoped that this series will fulfill its purpose of providing quick and easy access to critical information for the busy practitioner or trainee, and that it will assist pathologists in their routine practice of the specialty.

Saul Suster, MD
Professor and Chairman
Department of Pathology
Medical College of Wisconsin
Milwaukee, Wisconsin

Preface

The field of breast pathology has for decades attracted the attention of numerous health professionals including not only pathologists, medical oncologists, and surgeons, but general practitioners, residents, and medical students as well. Breast pathology is a dynamically developing field, and major progress has been achieved during recent decades with numerous important advances toward timely diagnoses and optimal treatments for breast cancer patients.

This book in the Demos Surgical Pathology Guides series has been designed to provide essential information by means of a concise, synoptic text addressing selected lesions including but not limited to those more commonly seen in routine practice. Nonetheless, traditional morphology, coupled with clinical data, has been emphasized, complementing each section chapter with as many photographs as possible, including macroscopic images. Diagnostic immunohistochemistry is mentioned under particular headings. Needless to say, this book is not intended as a comprehensive textbook of breast pathology, although we have sought to be as exhaustive as possible and in addition to the common entities, we have also included selected rare conditions, supplemented by literature citations. Our goal has been to provide a practical, rapid reference for the practitioner or trainee that will be a valuable tool for use in diagnosis or an efficient resource for review.

The Authors

Common Benign Conditions

1

FIBROCYSTIC CHANGES

PERIDUCTAL MASTITIS (DUCT ECTASIA)

FAT NECROSIS

SILICON MASTITIS

PREGNANCY/HORMONE-RELATED CHANGES

DIABETIC MASTOPATHY

ADENOSIS

SPECIAL TYPES OF ADENOSIS:
Sclerosing Adenosis
Microglandular Adenosis

Fibrocystic Changes

DEFINITION
- Fibrocystic changes (FCC) is a generic term indicating very frequent pathologic changes affecting the breast lobule and manifesting as combined cystic dilation of one or more gland units and increased fibrosis of the stroma, although their proportion may considerably vary.
- FCC are often associated with other pathologic conditions such as usual epithelial hyperplasia and adenosis.
- No longer used synonyms, that implied an underlying pathology, include fibrocystic disease, breast dysplasia, mazoplasia, fibroadenosis, and fibrous mastopathy. All these terms are either antiquated or inaccurate and should not be used in clinical practice.

CLINICAL FEATURES
- FCC are typically seen in premenopausal adult woman in the fourth and fifth decades. They are unusual in younger and postmenopausal women. Most common symptoms include premenopausal swelling of breast with pain and tenderness; however, their clinical presentation depends on the extent and size of FCC: on breast palpation, larger cysts are nontender, rubbery consolidations with smooth contours. Ruptured cyst may be associated with pain, secondary to lumen content leaking into the adjacent breast tissue and is likely to be responsible of mastodynia. Commonly, FCC may be totally asymptomatic.
- Mammographic films may show increased but nonhomogeneous density due to stromal fibrosis. It depends on overlapping profiles of smaller multiple cysts and/or the presence of larger, dominant cysts. Microcalcifications may be present, although not to the extent typically seen in proliferative diseases. Ultrasound demonstrates cysts and fibrosis.
- FCC represent hormonally mediated exaggeration of normal breast tissue. It is debatable whether gross cysts are associated with increased risk of cancer; however, the prevailing opinions negate such an association.

GROSS FEATURES
- In most cases, multiple, multifocal, and bilateral cysts surrounded by fibrosis are present. The cysts are smooth and tense. The cyst walls have a bluish to brown discoloration due to accumulated cellular and hematic material. The cyst fluid may be serous or granular depending on its chemical composition and cellularity.

MICROSCOPIC FEATURES
- The cyst wall is usually lined by large cuboidal to columnar cells often exhibiting a characteristic granular and eosinophilic cytoplasm with located nuclei; such cells are called apocrine cells (Figure 1-1). The chromatin is fine and nucleoli may be easily recognized. In classic cases, the cytoplasm has also fine PAS-positive glycolipid granules. Apocrine "snouts" may often be seen (Figure 1-2). Oxalate crystals may be found inside the cysts.

(continued)

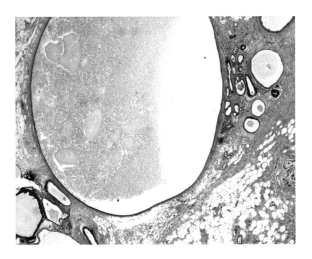

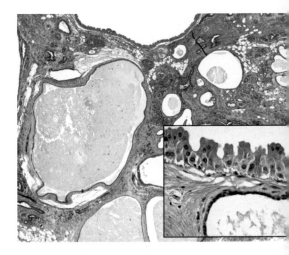

FIGURE 1-1
Fibrocystic changes (FCC). Panoramic view showing variably dilated ducts with macro- and microcyst formation lined by flattened epithelium often with apocrine changes. The larger cysts contain granular and mostly acellular serous-like material.

FIGURE 1-2
FCC. The intervening stroma has evidence of fibrosis and scattered inflammatory cells. Inset highlights apocrine cells: cytoplasm is granular to pink, luminal poles bulge into the lumina, and nuclei are round and even throughout.

Fibrocystic Changes *(continued)*

- The apocrine epithelium may also be arranged in small projections protruding into the cyst lumen (Figure 1-3). In a minor but sizable number of cases, a complex architectural arrangement is noted, with Roman-arch or cribriform patterns (Figure 1-4). Cytologic features, however, are maintained.
- Apocrine metaplasia may be diffuse or focal; it may also involve the epithelium of the lobules causing enlargement and distortion of one or more glandular units.
- The intervening stroma features scant, fibroblast-like cellularity in a loose or denser matrix. Variable collagenization may be seen in long-standing cases or if rupture has occurred.
- In other cases, an ordinary, flattened, nonmetaplastic epithelium may be seen alone or in combination with apocrine changes. The epithelial lining may also be absent due to on-going chronic inflammation. Periductal inflammation may be seen (Figure 1-5). In these cases, the association of lymphocytes, plasma cells and histiocytes, or granulation tissue indicates spillover of the cyst fluid.
- Cyst rupture may also be caused by invasive diagnostic procedures such as fine-needle aspiration or tru-cut biopsy.
- Epithelial detachment may be observed in some cases. In these cases, delicate strings of epithelial cells may be recognized within the cystic lumina.
- Proliferative changes may be intimately associated with FCC, although the relationship is unclear (Figure 1-6).

SPECIAL STUDIES
In contrast to periductal mastitis, silver stains do not demonstrate elastic fibers.

DIFFERENTIAL DIAGNOSIS
- Periductal mastitis/duct ectasia will be addressed in the next section. It should be re-minded that both the conditions may coexist.
- Minor dilation of terminal ducts should not be interpreted as FCC, although the thresh-old between simple ectasia and cyst is arbitrary; furthermore, sectioning artifacts may make the distinction difficult.
- Galactocele is a clinical differential diagnosis occurring in postlactation months due to condensed milk accumulated in the central breast. History of sudden lactation is often elicited when an inflamed cyst becomes symptomatic.
- Apocrine changes are not unique to FCC and may be observed in other benign breast entities, including adenosis, sclerosing adenosis, fibroadenoma, papilloma, radial scar, hamartoma as well as in otherwise normal gland units. Their significance is uncertain; however, larger cell size and nucleolar prominence of apocrine cells may raise the index of suspicion and suggest malignancy. Changes may be focal or diffuse. In situ and invasive carcinoma, either of lobular or ductal type, may also feature prominent apocrine features.

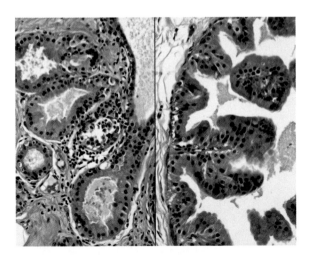

FIGURE 1-3
Apocrine epithelium may involve small duct units (left) or present as papillary configuration with delicate fibrovascular cores (right).

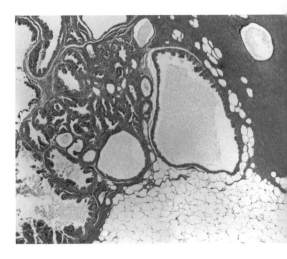

FIGURE 1-4
FCC showing extensive apocrine changes with mild proliferative features.

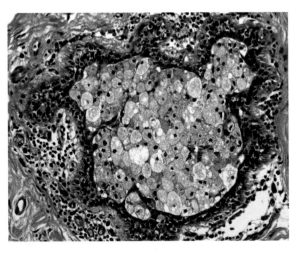

FIGURE 1-5
In FCC, ducts may show nonspecific chronic inflammation and luminal sloughing of histiocytic-like elements. Notice small, hyperchromatic nuclei and foamy cytoplasm.

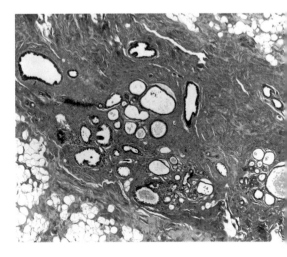

FIGURE 1-6
Panoramic view of FCC showing ductal proliferative changes. Apical snouts may be recognized.

Periductal Mastitis (Duct Ectasia)

DEFINITION
■ An extralobular disease usually affecting subareolar ductal structures. Also known as duct ectasia, a term emphasizing the dominant pathologic feature.
■ The cause is unknown, although anaerobic bacteria may be responsible. Cigarette smoking has also been implicated.
■ Some authors consider periductal mastitis to be a different condition from duct ectasia.

CLINICAL FEATURES
■ Although as much as 30% of women in their fifth to sixth decades may harbor microscopic changes compatible with periductal mastitis, clinical manifestations are seen in only a minority of cases.
■ Most patients are young adults, nonlactating women in their reproductive years. Past pregnancies and lactation may be predisposing factors, and suckling is a postulated triggering factor. Anecdotical cases in male patients have been reported as well.
■ Nipple retraction may be seen associated with either discharge or mass formation, mostly in older patients.
■ Routine mammograms may show images simulating carcinoma.

MICROSCOPIC FEATURES
■ A spectrum of microscopic features may be seen depending on the stage of the disease.
■ Initially, periductal chronic inflammation and progressive dilation of the affected duct are seen (Figure 1-7). Irregular cyst formation is associated with a decreased inflammatory component. Lumina content is initially serous-like then condensed. Foamy histiocytes and debris are commonly seen.
■ In advanced stages, periductal fibrosis is common (Figure 1-8) and may be responsible for nipple inversion.
■ In late stages, several changes may be noted, in particular abnormal dilatation of lumina; hence, the alternative designation of this condition as "duct ectasia" (Figures 1-9, 1-10, and 1-11). Lumina are plugged with proteinaceous-like material which distort the dilated duct profile. Periductal fibrosis may condense into sclerotic nodules with hyaline qualities bulging or obliterating the dilated spaces.
■ Linear or cast calcifications may be present and noticed on mammograms.
■ There is no associated epithelial hyperplasia. Apocrine metaplastia is uncommon.
■ Microscopic tissue changes are often paralleled by progressive damage of the periductal elastic membrane eventuating into near-total destruction in late stage.

(continued)

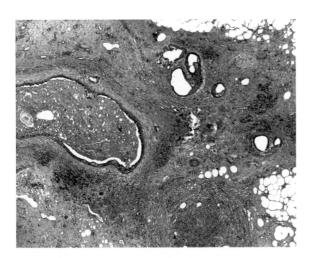

FIGURE 1-7
Periductal inflammation and duct dilation are present. Early changes show distortion of ducts due to active inflammation and periductal fibrosis.

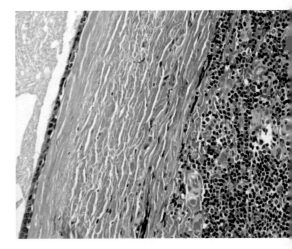

FIGURE 1-8
Periductal inflammation showing fibrosis and lymphomononuclear infiltrates.

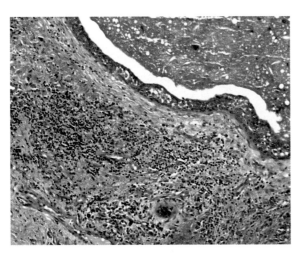

FIGURE 1-9
Closer view of an inflamed cystic duct showing inflammatory changes in the stroma subjacent to the epithelium. A frequent feature of mastitis is a dense, pink granular material resembling colostrum within the dilated lumina.

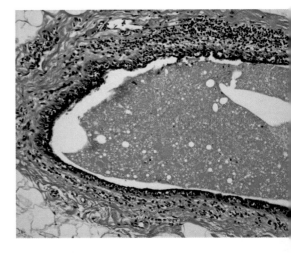

FIGURE 1-10
Duct ectasia/mastitis showing mild to moderate periductal inflammation with intraepithelial lymphocyte migration.

Periductal Mastitis (Duct Ectasia) *(continued)*

SPECIAL STUDIES
- ▪ Silver stains may be useful to demonstrate focal, often thickened residual of periductal elastic fibers.

DIFFERENTIAL DIAGNOSIS
- ▪ Although any cyst-forming lesion may enter the differential diagnosis, duct ectasia is the principal condition to be differentiated from periductal mastitis. Duct ectasia, that may be a different condition, usually affects older women, is considered an aging phenomenon, and does not have apparently a relationship to cigarette smoking or infection.
- ▪ Not infrequently, periductal mastitis and FCC coexist.
- ▪ As with any condition clinically characterized by nipple discharge, Paget disease is another important consideration in the differential diagnosis.

Periductal Mastitis (Duct Ectasia)

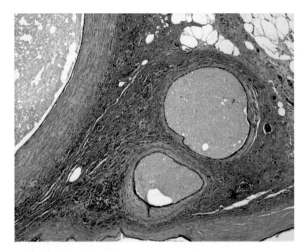

FIGURE 1-11
Chronic mastitis with fibrosis and
cystic ducts with flattened epithelium. These changes are usually seen
in late stage of the disease.

Fat Necrosis

DEFINITION
■ A relatively common disease of breast resulting from trauma such as motor vehicle accident or more often as a consequence of previous needle or surgical procedures. History of mammary reconstruction and radiotherapy for breast carcinoma is sometimes reported.

CLINICAL FEATURES
■ Fat necrosis may cause a suspicious painless, ill-defined palpable consolidation usually in the periareolar or superficial tissue of the breast. Nipple retraction is possible, although not very frequent.

■ Patient history is crucial for correct pathologic interpretation. When related to trauma, the lesion appears between 1 and 3 weeks after injury and may be associated with hematoma formation. The mean time for patients to present with a breast lump from the time of trauma is 68.5 weeks (range 3–208).

■ A broad range of image findings can be documented by means of mammography, breast ultrasound, and MRI, including spiculated opacities, multiple pleomorphic microcalcifications, dystrophic calcifications, cystic changes depending on the amount and extent of reparative fibrosis. In late stages, imaging may show features consistent with lipid cyst. Reparative changes may be represented by dystrophic calcifications or spiculated opacities.

PATHOLOGIC FEATURES
■ Grossly, fat necrosis appears as a consolidated area of hemorrhage, usually affecting the subcutaneous adipose tissue of the breast rather than the mammary parenchyma proper (Figure 1-12). Acute inflammatory changes dominate in early stages, followed by necrosis of adipose tissue, increased vascularization and infiltration by lymphocytes, and foamy histiocytes and fibroblasts (Figure 1-13).

■ Tissue debris are ultimately surrounded by epithelioid and multinucleated histiocytes associated with variable fibrous reparative changes (Figures 1-14 and 1-15).

■ Cystic degeneration may eventually ensue.

■ Degenerated erythrocytes within the fatty material released from necrotic adipocytes lead to conglomerations described in needle aspirates as "myospherulosis," considered cytologically diagnostic of fat necrosis.

■ Healed lesions are characterized by fibrous scarring associated with hemosiderin deposits.

DIFFERENTIAL DIAGNOSIS
■ Cyst rupture with content extravasation into the adjacent breast fat may result in clinical and pathologic changes difficult to discriminate from fat necrosis.

■ Consolidated, healed lesions may mimic infiltrating carcinoma clinically and on radiographic images.

■ History of trauma and/or breast surgery are crucial to correct pathologic interpretation.

■ Membranous fat necrosis is a cystic lesion with fine eosinophilic membrane and intracystic papillary-like projections of varying size that may mimic parasite cuticle.

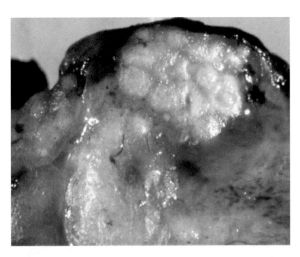

FIGURE 1-12
Gross specimen of fat necrosis showing irregular and confluent yellowish consolidations.

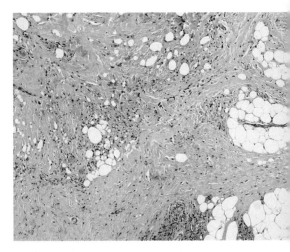

FIGURE 1-13
Fat necrosis showing liponecrosis, lipogranulomas, and fibrous scarring.

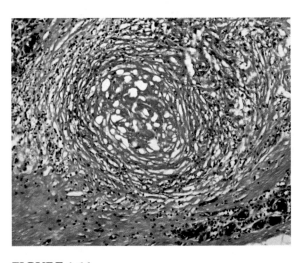

FIGURE 1-14
A focus of mammary liponecrosis associated with mild inflammation.

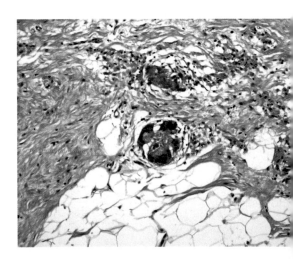

FIGURE 1-15
A high-power view of small lipogranulomas detailing confluent multinucleated histiocytes containing fat particles. A few mononuclear, epithelioid histiocytes are also present.

Silicone Mastitis

DEFINITION

■ An inflammatory condition of the breast secondary to silicone or silicone degradation products. Altered local immunity may be a favoring factor. Some case reports have documented the relationship between autoimmune diseases and silicone implants. However, several case-control studies have failed to show this association.

■ Malignant tumors including carcinoma and lymphoma of the breast have been reported in association with silicone implants; however, there is no evidence that extravasation of prosthetic material has carcinogenetic properties.

CLINICAL FEATURES

■ Silicone mastitis is characterized by painful induration, reddening, and increased pigmentation. Migrating nodules may be observed. In severe cases, draining sinuses may form.

■ Mammographic films show multiple nodular densities and may simulate carcinoma.

■ Hemorrhage with late hematoma formation may complicate silicon mastitis.

PATHOLOGIC FEATURES

■ The formation of a fibrous capsule around an implanted device in the breast is a normal event, comparable to a foreign body reaction elsewhere (Figure 1-16). It is microscopically characterized by an inner, synovial-like layer associated with scattered foreign body granulomatous reaction within a fibrous ground substance (Figures 1-17 and 1-18).

■ In silicone mastitis, a broad range of abnormal features may be seen depending on the amount of foreign substance leaked from the prosthetic device shell, and the extent and quality of inflammatory reaction. A lipogranulomatous inflammation is often seen with multinucleated giant cells engulfing oil-like material, fibroblastic activation, and histiocytic infiltration (Figures 1-19 and 1-20). Involvement of regional lymph nodes may be clinically noted with lipid-laden histiocytes and granuloma formation.

■ In severe cases, fat necrosis and tuberculoid-like reactions can be seen. Sclerosing and often disfiguring scarring may follow, requiring radical surgical intervention.

(continued)

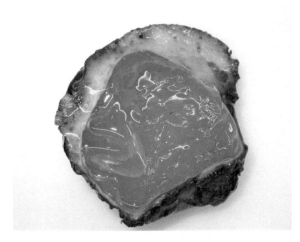

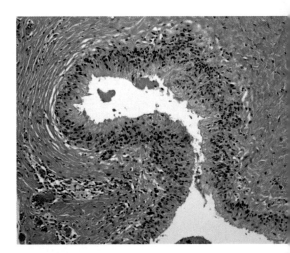

FIGURE 1-16
Gross specimen of silicone implant and adjacent breast tissue showing evidence of fibrous reaction and small cyst-like spaces filled with leaked prosthetic material (silicon jelly) (courtesy of Dr Jože Pižem, Ljubljana).

FIGURE 1-17
Fibrous pseudocapsule featuring palisading epithelioid histiocytes (the so-called synovial-like metaplasia) and fibrous scarring.

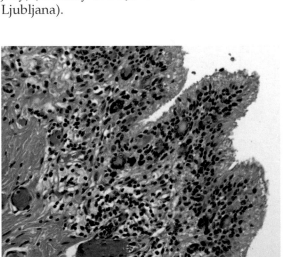

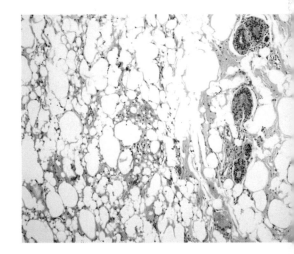

FIGURE 1-18
High-power magnification of inflammatory infiltrate in a case of silicon granuloma.

FIGURE 1-19
Breast tissue with scattered particles, representing leaked elastomere material, along with scant inflammatory cells.

Silicone Mastitis *(continued)*

DIFFERENTIAL DIAGNOSIS

■ Infection-related granulomatous mastitis requires clinical correlation and microbiological confirmation. Pathologic changes are not specific; tuberculous mastitis may present with draining tracts and often features caseating granulomas. Gomori methenamine silver and acid fast bacilli stains may assist in the initial microscopic evaluation.

■ Granulomatous lobular mastitis (the so-called Kessler-Wollock mastitis) is a rare condition of uncertain pathogenesis affecting young to young-adult women, clinically simulating carcinoma. Microscopically, it lacks caseating granuloma and lipid-laden cells.

■ Diabetic mastopathy may occasionally show a florid granulomatous reaction.

■ Sarcoid-like reaction has been documented in patients with breast cancer.

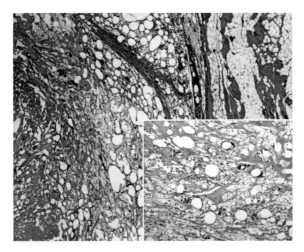

FIGURE 1-20
Silicon granuloma with numerous, confluent granulomas featuring mono- and multinucleated cells
associated with fibrous reaction.
The histiocytes are filled with foreign
material.

Pregnancy/Hormone-Related Changes

DEFINITION
■ A spectrum of physiologic changes in the breast secondary to pregnancy, including lactation. Comparable changes may be seen in patients treated with exogenous hormones or with increased susceptibility to endogenous hormones.

MICROSCOPIC FEATURES
■ Early pregnancy-related changes are evident during the second month of gestation and include enlargement and increased pigmentation of nipple and areola.
■ Microscopically, early pregnancy-related changes feature mild enlargement of the terminal duct lobular units along with the formation of new units (the so-called pregnancy-related adenosis); supranuclear vacuolation may not be prominent (Figures 1-21 and 1-22).
■ During the second trimester of gestation cytoplasmic secretion is more evident and precedes the well-developed lactational stage seen in the third trimester characterized by prominent lipid-laden cytoplasm, lumina distension with accumulation of eosinophilic secretion (colostrum), and decreased interlobular stroma with back-to-back arranged lobular units.
■ Other changes also include hobnail and apocrine cells lining the lactating acini (Arias-Stella phenomenon). Nuclei can be hyperchromatic (Figures 1-23 and 1-24).
■ Comparable changes may be seen in nonlactating breast; however, these changes are usually partial.

(*continued*)

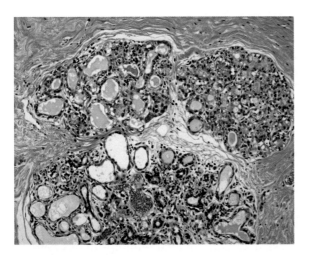

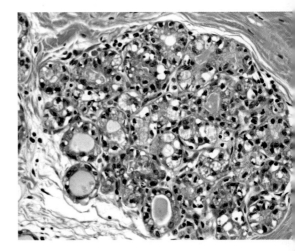

FIGURE 1-21
Lobular units showing the so-called pregnancy-related adenosis, including hyperplastic changes and cytoplasmic vacuolization. Scattered lymphoid cells may be recognized.

FIGURE 1-22
High-power magnification of Figure 1-21. The lumina contain eosinophilic material.

Pregnancy/Hormone-Related Changes *(continued)*

CLINICAL FEATURES

■ Residual lactation-related changes may be seen in women up to 1 year after delivery.

■ In nonpregnant patients, lactation-type changes may be related to estrogen therapy or contraceptive pills. However, in a small percentage of cases, there is no clinical evidence of exogenous hormone administration. An increased lobular susceptibility to endogenous estrogen has been claimed for these cases.

■ Pregnancy may induce modifications in preexisting or concomitant breast lesions. Some lactating adenomas probably represent fibroadenoma undergoing cellular and stromal gestational changes, although most lactational adenomas are focal, nonneoplastic adeno-matous hyperplasia (ie, the hyperplasia of pregnancy is uneven and may grow more in one area than the other.) It is also thought that most lactational adenomas regress sponta-neously after delivery. Infarction of lactational adenoma is a well-known, clinically acute event characterized by pain and a tender mass. Infarction can be partial or total and may be associated with ischemic events in the nontumoral conditions.

■ Similar microscopic features have been described in males treated with hormones for prostatic carcinoma.

DIFFERENTIAL DIAGNOSIS

■ In nonlactating, nonpregnant women, the lesions may be very focal and may be related to hormonal, antipsychotic, or antihypertensive treatment or without any obvious cause.

■ Lobular neoplasia, glycogen-rich carcinoma, metastatic clear cell carcinoma, or signet-ring cell carcinoma may be simulated by pregnancy or hormone-related changes featur-ing extensive clear cells.

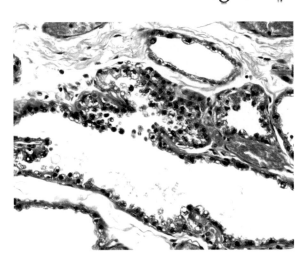

FIGURE 1-23
Nuclear hobnailing is often seen in late pregnancy or during lactation.

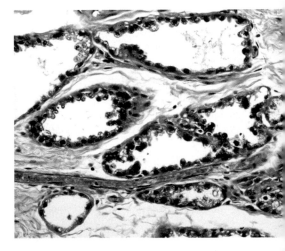

FIGURE 1-24
Hyperchromatic nuclei are also commonly seen in pregnancy or during exogenous hormone administration.

Diabetic Mastopathy

DEFINITION
■ An inflammatory fibrosing condition of the breast most often associated with long history of type I diabetes, thought to represent an abnormal local immune reaction.

■ Not commonly, diabetic mastopathy changes may be seen in patients with type II diabetes as well as in nondiabetic subjects. Sporadic cases have been reported in males and in patients suffering from autoimmune diseases such as arthritis, Sjogren syndrome or chronic thyroiditis, and some other autoimmune diseases.

■ Foci of similar changes adjacent to breast carcinoma have been described as well.

CLINICAL FEATURES
■ Diabetic mastopathy may present with palpable subareolar lumps in pre- or sometimes perimenopausal women. In males, it can simulate gynecomastia.

■ Diabetic mastopathy can be seen mammographically, and recurrences may be seen in about one-fourth of cases.

PATHOLOGIC FEATURES
■ Unilateral nodular, palpable consolidations of the subareolar breast are most often seen. The microscopic dominant features include infiltration of inflammatory cells within a fibrous or sclerotic keloid-like stroma, the latter accounting for the sustained tissue consistency. In rare cases, the diabetic mastopathy may be bilateral.

■ The inflammatory cell population is composed mostly of small round lymphocytes, showing perilobular, perivascular, and periductal arrangement; hence, the "lymphocytic lobulitis with fibrosis" designation is adopted by several authors (Figure 1-25). Scattered plasma cells and neutrophils may also be seen.

■ The degree of periductular/perilobular inflammation may be moderate to heavy as to obscure the involved lobular units. Small vessels may be obliterated by dense lymphoid infiltrates as well (Figures 1-26 and 1-27).

■ Scattered or clusters of plump, epithelioid fibroblast-like cells may be documented in the stroma (Figure 1-28). The atypical stromal cells exhibit strong positivity for CD10.

■ B-lymphocytes apparently predominate and B-cell lymphoepithelial complex described; however, there is apparently no increased risk of malignant lymphoma in association with diabetic mastopathy.

DIFFERENTIAL DIAGNOSIS
■ Breast fibromatosis may be associated with increased, keloid-like collagenization, although generally not to the extent seen in diabetic mastopathy. Furthermore, epithelioid fibroblasts are not observed in fibromatosis and inflammatory lesions are not its feature.

■ The lymphoid periductal infiltrate may be difficult to evaluate in frozen sections since it may simulate infiltrating lobular carcinoma.

■ Diabetic mastopathy may occasionally show florid granulomatous reaction.

■ In nondiabetic lobular mastitis, stromal fibrosis is less pronounced, there is less lobular atrophy, and epithelioid fibroblasts are rarely seen.

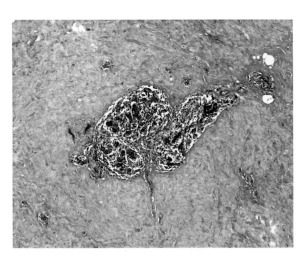

FIGURE 1-25
Diabetic mastopathy. Discrete lymphoid infiltration of a lobule within a sclerotic stroma.

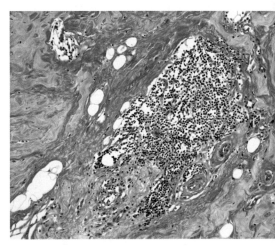

FIGURE 1-26
Diabetic mastopathy. In this case, the glandular units have been obliterated by the inflammatory infiltrate.

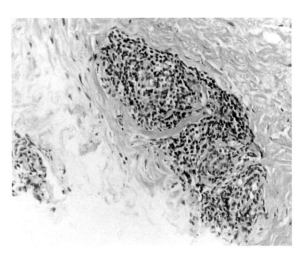

FIGURE 1-27
Diabetic mastopathy. The inflammatory cells show periductal and perivascular arrangement.

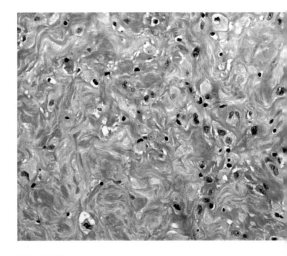

FIGURE 1-28
Diabetic mastopathy. Stromal cells of probable myofibroblastic origin exhibiting a relatively large size and epithelioid qualities. The ground substance is either fibrous or densely sclerotic.

Adenosis

DEFINITION

■ A descriptive, nondiagnostic term referring to an organized, benign proliferation of the terminal duct lobular unit of the breast that may or may not produce a palpable mass. It may also be seen in pregnancy.

■ Special variants such as microglandular adenosis and sclerosing adenosis have enough clinical and pathologic connotations and deserve attention under separate headings.

■ The so-called blunt duct adenosis is sometimes a synonym for columnar cell lesions that may be related to future neoplasia.

■ Adenosis is not associated with an increased risk for subsequent breast carcinoma.

CLINICAL FEATURES

■ Depending on the extent of hyperplastic changes, adenosis may or may not be palpable.

■ When it has larger size, the designation of "adenosis tumor" is often used. Adenosis tumor can be clearly palpable and may simulate a fibroadenoma clinically and on radiographic images.

■ Dystrophic microcalcifications in adenosis may be documented on screening mammograms.

MICROSCOPIC FEATURES

■ Low-power examination shows fairly round and well-defined nodules composed of enlarged tubular units that are often seen surrounding a terminal duct (Figure 1-29).

■ The hyperplastic tubules may have open lumina with a distorted or angulated outline and are often generally separated by a discrete amount of fibrous connective tissue comparable to that of the normal breast lobule (Figures 1-30 and 1-31).

■ The proportion between the glandular and stromal component varies within the same case, although epithelial hyperplasia tends to predominate.

■ A dual cell population is constantly present in the hyperplastic glands, ie, an outer, basal myoepithelial and a luminal, inner epithelial layer. The basal cells rest on a PAS-positive basement membrane and may be recognized in virtue of their smaller size, clear cytoplasm, flattened nuclei, and immunoreactivity to basal antigens, including cytokeratin 5, p63, and CD10. The luminal cells are either cuboidal or cylindrical and have more stainable cytoplasm or cyplasmic extrusion.

(continued)

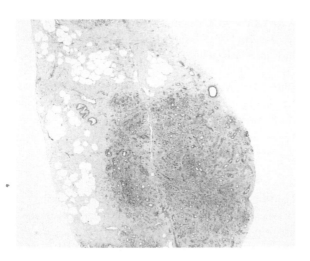

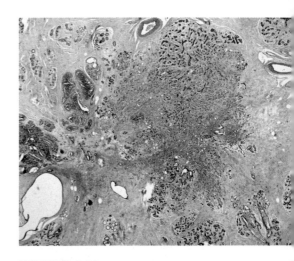

FIGURE 1-29
Adenosis. Panoramic view showing disorderly arranged gland units along with fibrous changes. The cellular area retains a lobular configuration and should not be confused with cancer.

FIGURE 1-30
A poorly defined focus of adenosis is adjacent to a focus of usual duct hyperplasia (left), along with some peripheral dilation of lumina. At this magnification, patent or collapsed tubular units may be noted.

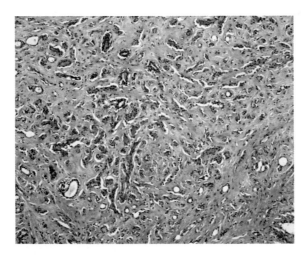

FIGURE 1-31
Pronounced gland distortion is seen with some tubular arrangements like so-called tubular adenosis.

Adenosis *(continued)*

■ Adenosis is very often seen in association with fibrocystic disease as well as in combination with special types of adenosis such as blunt duct adenosis (Figure 1-32), adenomyoepithelial adenosis (Figure 1-33) or microglandular adenosis (see below), and nodular adenosis.

■ Cellular lesions are also known as "florid adenosis." Mitotic figures may be seen, but they are not atypical and not associated with other features of malignancy.

■ Involvement by proliferative epithelial changes proper, including usual and atypical ductal hyperplasia, may be seen in breast adenosis. Association with atypical lobular hyperplasia and lobular carcinoma, however, is more common.

DIFFERENTIAL DIAGNOSIS

■ The main differential diagnosis is well differentiated (tubular type) infiltrating ductal carcinoma: criteria favoring adenosis are the organoid arrangement, a dual cell population and a variable amount of intervening stroma of fibrous type featuring bland fibroblasts, and a loosely textured ground substance. Infiltrating carcinoma, on the other hand, is associated with a destructive growth pattern, lacks a dual cell population, and has a nonspecialized, often hypocellular, desmoplastic stroma.

■ Tubular adenosis, a rare special type of adenosis, may also mimic infiltrating ductal carcinoma and microglandular adenosis.

■ Special stains for myoepithelial cells may be useful to distinguish adenosis from infiltrating carcinoma. Estrogen-receptor immunostaining may decorate scattered luminal cells in adenosis; on the other hand, cancer cells usually exhibit the "all or none" reaction pattern, ie, they are all-positive or all-negative for estrogen receptors.

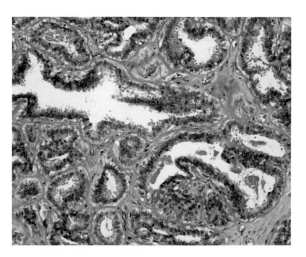

FIGURE 1-32
Blunt duct adenosis. The ducts are
dilated and show variable degree
of proliferative activity. A dual cell
population with bland nuclei may
be recognized: basal, myoepithelial
cells have clear cytoplasm, whereas
luminal cells are either cuboidal,
columnar, or flattened. The intervening stroma is also increased with scattered fibroblastoid cells.

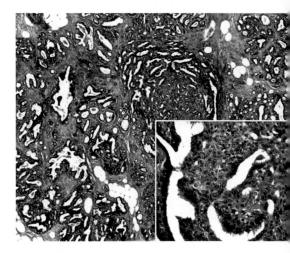

FIGURE 1-33
Adenomyoepithelial adenosis.
In this case, there is a marked
accompanying proliferation of
myoid elements that may focally
(inset) mimic an adeno myoepithelioma.
The glands are relatively enlarged
and show proliferative changes.

Special Types of Adenosis:
Sclerosing Adenosis

DEFINITION
- A lobular benign proliferation of deformed ductular/acinar elements with variable components of a sclerotic stroma. Scattered stromal and intraluminal calcifications are often seen.
- Due to its firm consistency, ill-defined nodule formation, and increased cellularity, sclerosing adenosis is considered a potential mimicker of infiltrating carcinoma.
- There are conflicting results as to the subsequent risk of cancer following sclerosing adenosis, ranging from no significant to slightly increased, depending on the presence of associated atypical epithelial hyperplasia.

CLINICAL FEATURES
- Often a palpable breast lesion occurring in reproductive ages and perimenopausal years and often associated with abnormal mammographic features including an ill-defined opacity and microcalcifications.

MICROSCOPIC FEATURES
- A lobulocentric lesion with haphazard arrangement of epithelial and myoepithelial cells with a variable fibrous ground substance. Increased cellularity is generally seen in the center of the lesion and features as collapsed aggregates with no patent lumina (Figure 1-34).
- Spectrum changes ranging from more cellular lesions to a sclerotic phase may be often noted. Cellular sclerosing adenosis characteristically features more myoid and spindle cells (Figure 1-35).
- Perineurial and intravascular growth should not be considered as a microscopic evidence of malignancy, especially if all the other features of sclerosing adenosis are present.
- Apocrine changes may be seen.
- As in common adenosis, a dual cell population is constantly present in sclerosing adenosis, ie, that is an outer, a basal myoepithelial, and a luminal epithelial layer.
- Sclerosing adenosis may undergo important changes in pregnancy and in situations associated with physiological or pathological hormone unbalances, including repeated pregnancies, lactation suppression, ovarian malfunction, etc.
- It may be seen in association with the FCC.
- Sclerosing adenosis may be rarely seen in sentinel lymph nodes.

(continued)

Special Types of Adenosis:
Sclerosing Adenosis

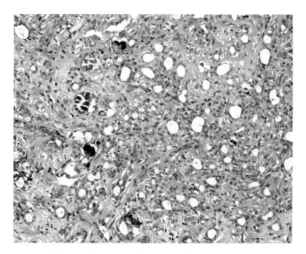

FIGURE 1-34
High-power view of adenosis
showing a mixture of haphazardly
arranged and distorted tubuloglandular structures. Microcalcifications
are often seen.

Special Types of Adenosis:
Sclerosing Adenosis (continued)

DIFFERENTIAL DIAGNOSIS

■ The main differential diagnosis is classic, infiltrating lobular carcinoma: the peculiar growth pattern of sclerosing adenosis described above should prompt its recognition. However, in core needle biopsy, the overall architecture assessment may not be as accurate as in lumpectomy specimens, and closely clustered ductules and acini may be mistaken for malignancy.

■ Because of its gross appearance and haphazard cell composition, sclerosing adenosis may be difficult to distinguish from invasive carcinoma in frozen sections submitted for intraoperative consultation.

■ A dual cell population of epithelial and myoepithelial cells is not seen in invasive lobular carcinoma. Haphazard admixture of apocrine cells is also not expected in invasive lobular carcinoma.

■ On the other hand, the one or two-cell filing microscopic pattern seen in infiltrating lobular carcinoma is not seen in sclerosing adenosis.

■ Sclerosing adenosis may be colonized by ductal or lobular carcinoma in situ.

Special Types of Adenosis:
Sclerosing Adenosis

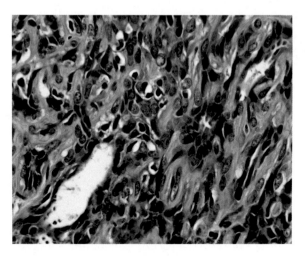

FIGURE 1-35
High-power view detailing spindle
cells with myoid qualities.

Special Types of Adenosis:
Microglandular Adenosis

DEFINITION
■ An uncommon form of nonlobulocentric hyperplasia of acinar-like units often resulting in an ill-defined and palpable lesion.
■ It is debated whether microglandular adenosis is a precancerous condition.

CLINICAL FEATURES
■ Due to its size, on average 3–5 cm, microglandular adenosis is an alarming clinical finding.

MICROSCOPIC FEATURES
■ The salient microscopic feature is a haphazard increase in small, round uniform tubular units with open lumina containing acid and neutral mucopolysaccharidic substances positive for PAS and Alcian Blue stains (Figure 1-36).
■ Glandular aggregates are poorly defined and may be documented within the normal breast, the mammary adipose tissue, or adjacent skeletal muscle, giving the false impression of an infiltrating ductal carcinoma (Figure 1-37).
■ The proliferating acinar units are composed of single layers of cuboidal to flattened epithelial cells. Myoepithelial cell layers are, by definition, absent (Figure 1-38).
■ The epithelial cells are positive for keratins. However, they are negative for endomysial autoantibody (EMA), estrogen, and myoepithelial markers (Figure 1-39).
■ In some cases, the lesion may progress through atypical microglandular adenosis (MA) to in situ or invasive carcinoma.

DIFFERENTIAL DIAGNOSIS
■ Tubular carcinoma is the main consideration since both the lesions display a remarkable infiltrative pattern and low-grade nuclei, yet microglandular adenosis is composed of fairly round to oval tubules and lacks the scar-like stroma of tubular carcinoma; the latter often features angulated rather than round acinar structures.
■ Tubular carcinoma has often associated foci of ductal carcinoma in situ of cribriform pattern.
■ Special stains for myoepithelial cells are of no help since both the conditions lack a basal layer. Estrogen receptor and EMA are usually diffusely and strongly positive in tubular carcinoma and negative in microglandular adenosis. These two markers are helpful in distinguishing microglandular adenosis from carcinoma.

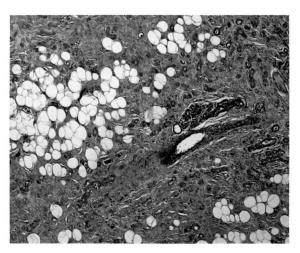

FIGURE 1-36
Microglandular adenosis. Disorderly small duct units lacking lobular arrangement dissecting a variably sclerotic stroma.

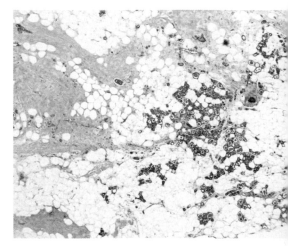

FIGURE 1-37
Microglandular adenosis. The tubular units are lined by a single layer of polygonal cells. Lumina are round, patent, and often contain eosinophilic secretion.

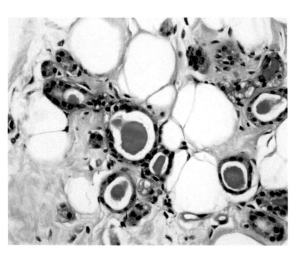

FIGURE 1-38
Microglandular adenosis. The luminal secretion may have dense and eosinophilic qualities.

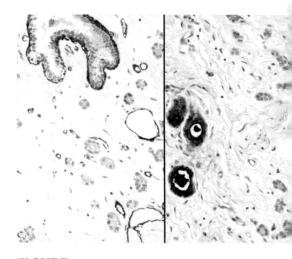

FIGURE 1-39
Microglandular adenosis. Note the lack of a myoepithelial cell layer (left, smooth muscle actin stain). The epithelial cells are negative for EMA (right) in contrast to normal mammary glands that react positively.

Chapter 1: Common Benign Conditions   *31*

Proliferative and Preinvasive Epithelial Lesions

2

Usual Ductal Hyperplasia

DEFINITION
■ Also known as epitheliosis, moderate hyperplasia, florid hyperplasia, fenestrated epitheliosis, ductal papillomatosis, etc. Usual ductal hyperplasia (UDH), according to the WHO scheme, is a proliferative disorder carrying a small though definitive risk of breast cancer, about 1.5–2 folds.

CLINICAL FEATURES
■ There are no specific radiologic findings in UDH. However, it may be associated with a clinically palpable nodule and glandular opacities with clustered calcifications in mammograms.

GROSS FEATURES
■ UDH does not have specific findings on gross examination. It is usually part of other benign and malignant proliferative breast diseases.
■ Macroscopic examination of breast specimens shows variable tissue consolidation depending on the extent of the changes within the mammary gland. On a cut section, UDH areas appear lucent, gray white, ill defined. Rarely, UDH may have extensive microcalcifications. In these cases, the consolidated areas are gritty on sectioning.

MICROSCOPIC FEATURES
■ Low-power assessment shows abnormally distended termino-lobular duct units showing variable cellularity. Epithelial cells are arranged around clear spaces classically designated as "fenestrations" forming irregular bridges (Figure 2-1). Fenestrations in UDH show characteristically uneven silhouettes and are most often peripheral, branching, or arch-shaped (Figure 2-2). In central parts, the proliferating cells may show streaming pattern of growth. However in solid UDH, fenestrations may be obscured by the proliferating cells or be only barely recognized as focal slit-like spaces (Figure 2-3).
■ High-magnification evaluation of UDH shows irregular size and shape of proliferating cells, ranging from oval to spindle or twisted nuclei (Figures 2-4 and 2-5). Cell orientation is also variable. Because of increased cellularity, nuclei often overlap and may impart a syncytial pattern to the proliferation, especially when they fill the duct lumen. Cell membranes are difficult to discern. Apocrine and myoepithelial cells may be a part of proliferating cell population.

(continued)

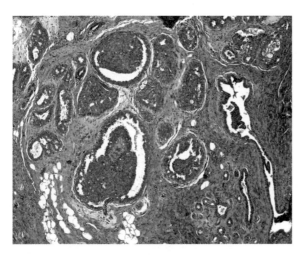

FIGURE 2-1
Usual duct hyperplasia (UDH).
Disorderly arranged solid cellular
nests partially obliterate the duct
lumina.

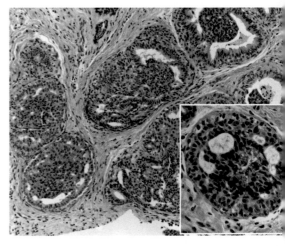

FIGURE 2-2
Fenestrations of UDH are variable,
peripheral, and branching.
Microcalcifications are often seen
(inset).

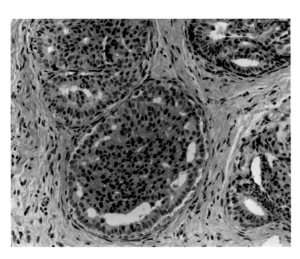

FIGURE 2-3
High-power view detailing florid
hyperplastic changes and peripheral
fenestration.

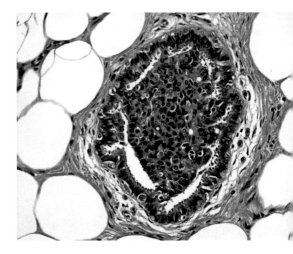

FIGURE 2-4
UDH. There is a haphazard mixture
of ductal and myoepithelial cells.
Nuclei are of variable size and shape.

Usual Ductal Hyperplasia *(continued)*

◼ Fenestrations may be empty or optically clear. However, not infrequently, they may be filled with foamy histiocytes (Figure 2-6) that, when extensive, simulate comedonecrosis. It is important to remember that cell necrosis is not a feature of UDH. The presence of focal necrotic spots, usually in larger lesions because of a poor vascular supply or previous invasive procedures, however, does not preclude a diagnosis of UDH as long as the other features are present. Squamous metaplastic changes may be seen, as reparative changes, following tissue necrosis.

◼ Scattered lymphoid elements may be recognized within the proliferating epithelium or may shed into the ductular lumina.

◼ Mitotic figures as well as prominent nucleoli are not part of the spectrum of microscopic changes, although they may be seen occasionally.

◼ High-molecular weight keratins show a mosaic staining pattern. Myoepithelial cells are highlighted by means of an anti-p63 antibody.

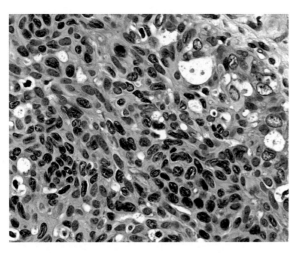

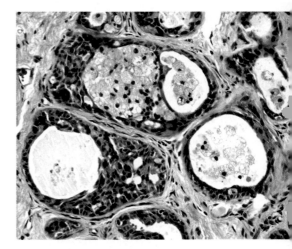

FIGURE 2-5
Florid duct hyperplasia. Ductal and myoepithelial cells often becoming spindly. Although some nuclei have finely dispersed chromatin and may raise the index of suspicion, the combined presence of different cell shape and size, uneven patent spaces, and the absence of a brisk mitotic activity and necrosis exclude (or speak against) a diagnosis of malignancy.

FIGURE 2-6
UDH featuring foamy macrophages.

Atypical Ductal Hyperplasia

DEFINITION
■ Atypical ductal hyperplasia (ADH) of the breast, or DIN 1b according to the WHO classification, may be defined as proliferative lesions showing intermediate features between UDH and low-grade ductal carcinoma in situ (LG-DCIS) at the architectural and cytological level and extent of disease.

■ Under different perspectives, it may be also defined as (a) an "incomplete" form of low-grade DCIS or (b) as a lesion harboring all features of LG-DCIS *but* of limited extent, ie, a small LG-DCIS. No consensus has been reached yet, among breast pathology experts, in regard of the quantitative criteria enabling the distinction between ADH and LG-DCIS.

■ It has been proposed to include within the ADH category, lesions measuring up to 2 mm in aggregate or involving two distinct duct spaces.

■ ADH carries a definite increased relative risk (4–5 folds) for developing subsequent breast cancer. The risk involves both breasts and may show any type and grade.

■ ADH documented in core needle biopsy specimens is generally regarded as an indication for further surgical evaluation.

CLINICAL FEATURES
ADH does not have specific clinical or mammographic features. However, it may be associated with clinically palpable nodules such as papillomas and radial sclerosing lesions. Rarely, clustered calcifications may be noted in mammograms.

GROSS FEATURES
■ ADH is not commonly detected grossly. A palpable breast mass may be detected, when associated with other breast lesions.

MICROSCOPIC FEATURES
■ An abnormal expansion of the duct units is characteristically observed at a panoramic view (Figure 2-7). Fenestrations are commonly recognized; however, cell bridges may lack the plasticity seen in UDH and are focally round or "punched-out" (Figure 2-8). The epithelial cells may also been arranged in micropapillae. Other accepted criterion is <2 mm low-grade lesion even if the ducts are entirely involved. A portion of the involved gland unit usually features UDH.

■ On a closer view, monotonous, round cells with discernible cell membrane and round nuclei, comparable to those seen in LG-DCIS, are observed (Figures 2-9 and 2-10).

■ Since the differences between ADH and LG-DCIS appear only "quantitative," the level of interobserver agreement is low. Questions have been raised whether ADH should be distinguished from low-grade DCIS, considering that cells within ADH have been demonstrated to be clonal, hence neoplastic. However, compelling evidence from clinical follow-up investigations indicates that ADH and DCIS should be still considered distinct. Disagreements among observers may be reduced using proposed criteria by Page as well as Tavassoli.

■ High-molecular weight keratins show decreased or absent staining pattern. Anti-p63 antibody decorates the basal layer of myoepithelial cells.

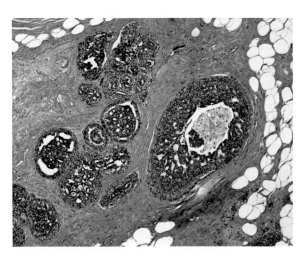

FIGURE 2-7
Atypical ductal hyperplasia (ADH).
Ducts are abnormally distended by
proliferating epithelial cells. The
features lie between UDH and cribriform ductal carcinoma in situ (DCIS).

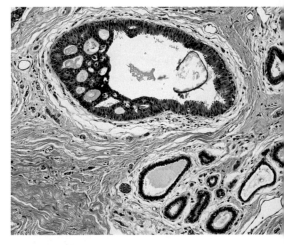

FIGURE 2-8
Partial involvement of the duct with
DCIS-like lesion with punched-out
spaces. These changes, however, are
not sufficient for the designation
of DCIS.

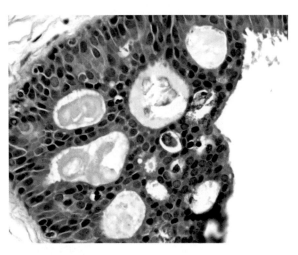

FIGURE 2-9
High-power magnification of
Figure 2-2 detailing a relative mo-
notonous appearance of nuclei that
are predominantly round to oval.
Microcalcifications are evident.

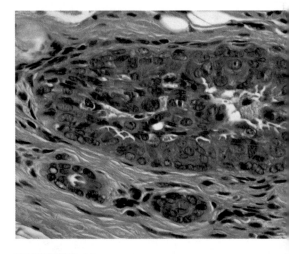

FIGURE 2-10
ADH showing barely recognizable
open, slit-like spaces between proliferating epithelial cells with round
to oval nuclei. Small nucleoli may be
recognized.

Columnar Cell Lesions

DEFINITION

■ A heterogeneous group of lesions involving the terminal duct lobular units and lined by epithelial cells exhibiting "columnar" features. A broad spectrum of proliferative changes, ranging from minimal or no atypia to high-grade cytoarchitectural disorder akin to DCIS, has been reported.

■ Columnar cell changes (CCC) have been known for a long time, and the lack of precise understanding of these lesions has resulted in a confused, often nonreproducible terminology.

■ The frequent association of CCC with mammographically detected microcalcifications has increased the practical significance of these lesions and led to a critical reappraisal of the subject, eventuating in a more organic and practical classification scheme.

■ CCC with cytologic atypia are referred as flat epithelial atypia (FEA).

CLINICAL FEATURES

■ Lack of adequate follow-up studies prevents conclusions to support a relationship between columnar cell lesions (CCC, columnar cell hyperplasia [CCH], FEA) and the subsequent risk of infiltrating carcinoma. Yet, microscopic (similar cytologic features, coexistent lesions, comparable immunophenotypes) molecular genetic and clinical data suggest that FEA is probably akin to LG-DCIS and should be cautiously treated with local excision.

GROSS FEATURES

■ Columnar cell lesions do not show specific macroscopic features. However, these lesions are often associated with fibrocystic changes.

MICROSCOPIC FEATURES

■ Simple columnar cell lesions are characterized by variably dilated ductal units lined by a single row of juxtaposed tall cells featuring elongated nuclei (Figure 2-11). The lumina may have tortuous profiles or be round attaining the size of a small cyst, which often contain a granular secretion. Microcalcifications are present though not constantly (Figure 2-12). The epithelial cells have eosinophilic cytoplasm and bland nuclei composed of fine chromatin with inconspicuous nucleoli (Figure 2-13). Cell protrusions within the lumina (apical snouts or blebs) are usually recognized (Figure 2-14). The intervening stroma is composed of fibroblast-like cells and may be loose or fibrotic. The lesions typically exhibit organoid pattern often with prominent myoepithelial layer and intracanalicular stromal protrusions.

■ Actively proliferating CCC are divided into two distinct categories: CCH and FEA.

(continued)

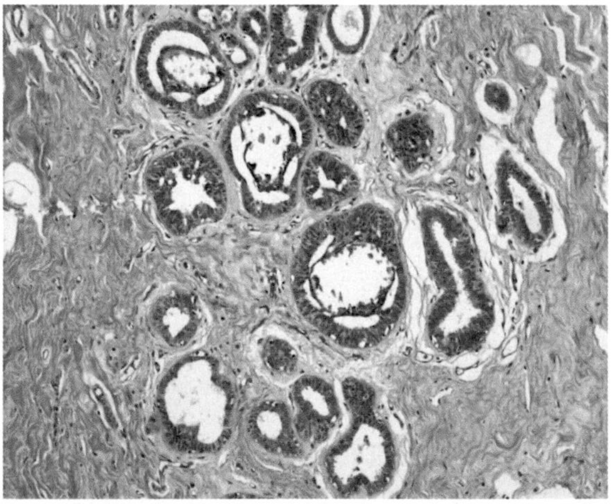

FIGURE 2-11
Simple columnar cell lesions featuring small cystic spaces lined by tall columnar cells.

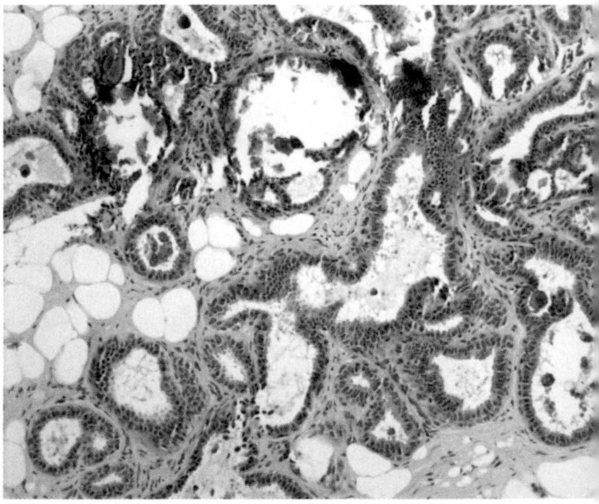

FIGURE 2-12
Phosphate-rich microcalcifications may dominate the microscopic features, although they are not always seen in columnar cell lesions.

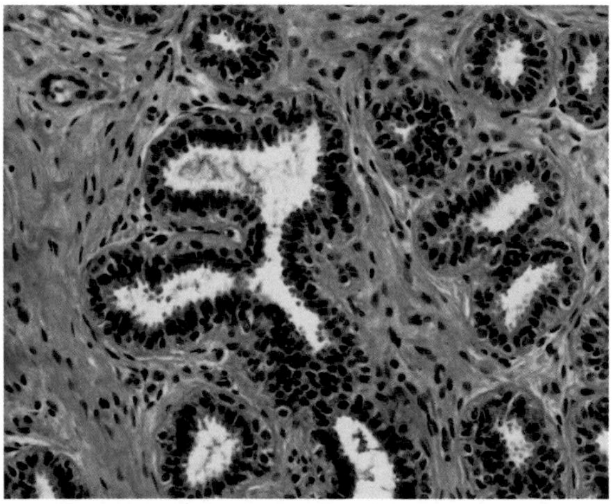

FIGURE 2-13
Columnar cell changes (CCC). A dual cell population may be recognized with luminal, tall cells resting on a layer of basal myoepithelial cells.

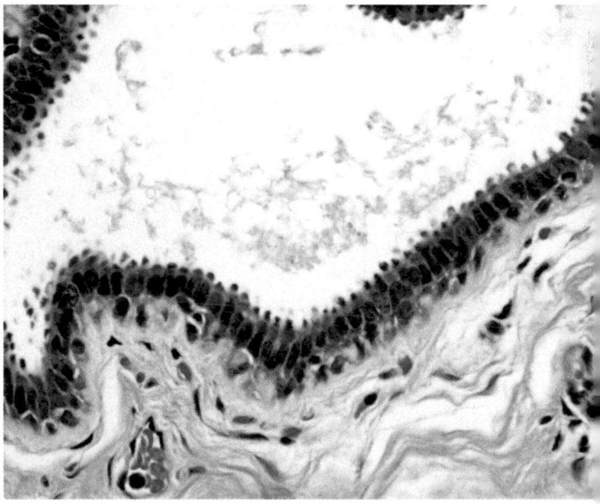

FIGURE 2-14
High-power view of CCC detailing the characteristic cytoplasmic snouts of the luminal cells and the monotonous bland appearance of their nuclei.

Columnar Cell Lesions (*continued*)

■ CCH characteristically has more than two cell layers, and this increased stratification of columnar cells is associated with more evident apical snouts, increased secretions, and prominent luminal microcalcifications. "Tufting" may be noticed; however, the cells of CCH have a slight variation in size and shape, nuclei are uniform with little or no atypia, and nucleoli are not prominent (Figure 2-15).

■ FEA or CCH with atypia features usually one, sometimes more layers of cuboidal to columnar cells having nonpolar, round rather than oval nuclei (Figure 2-16). The dilated lumina have dense granular material and often contain microcalcifications. Apical snouts/blebs may be prominent (Figure 2-17). FEA is virtually comparable to "clinging carcinoma," the microscopic entity originally described by Azzopardi and included in the spectrum of DCIS. FEA is generally positive for estrogen and progesterone receptors. In the WHO scheme, FEA is under the DIN1a heading.

■ FEA is seen with increased frequency in association with tubular carcinoma and with other intraepithelial and lobular neoplasia.

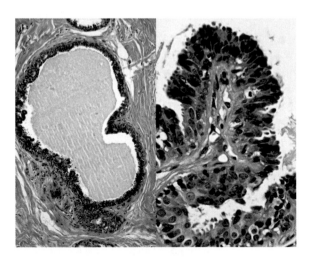

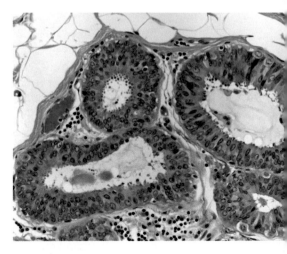

FIGURE 2-15
Columnar cell hyperplasia. Epithelial cell stratification, small papillary projections within the lumen, and nuclear pleomorphism.

FIGURE 2-16
Flat epithelial atypia (FEA). Cells are in single or pseudostratified layer and show usually nonpolar nuclei that are either round or tall.

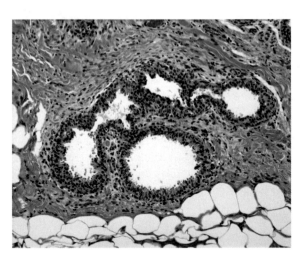

FIGURE 2-17
FEA. Apical snouts are prominent.

Ductal Carcinoma In Situ

DEFINITION
■ DCIS, also known as intraductal carcinoma, or DIN 3 represents a malignant proliferation of epithelial cells confined to the basement membrane of the ductal-lobular system. It is considered a precursor, although not obligate, of infiltrating carcinoma.
■ DCIS has different medical presentations and different microscopic phenotypes. These clinicopathological diversities reflect the variable biological potential and entail a number of management issues as well.

CLINICAL FEATURES
■ DCIS may present as palpable lesions. The most common presentation, however, is microcalcifications at the time of screening mammography.
■ The microcalcifications may be granular and low-density calcifications (most often seen in LG-DCIS), or linear, high-density branching or "casting" pleomorphic (observed in high-grade ductal carcinoma in situ, HG-DCIS).

GROSS FEATURES
■ Small or focal lesions may have inconspicuous macroscopic features. Lesions that have spread to the entire lobular unit appear as scattered, ill-defined gray white consolidations that may or may not express necrotic material (comedonecrosis) on light pressure (Figure 2-18).

MICROSCOPIC FEATURES
■ LG-DCIS, or DIN 1c, shows increased proliferation of neoplastic ductal cells arranged either in cribriform, papillary, or rarely solid architecture (Figure 2-19). A honeycomb pattern may be apparent. The round cell nuclei are centrally placed and have a monotonous appearance (Figure 2-20).
■ When a cribriform pattern is present, the cell population is evenly distributed around distinct oval to circular lumina. Compared to fenestrations of UDH or ADH, sharply delimited ("punched out"), of comparable size, and evenly spaced within the enlarged gland unit are observed in DCIS. Trabecular bridges or bars lack the pliability of UDH and are often composed of one or two cell layers with nuclei perpendicular to cribriform lumina.
■ A micropapillary or frank papillary pattern may be seen (Figures 2-21 and 2-22).

(continued)

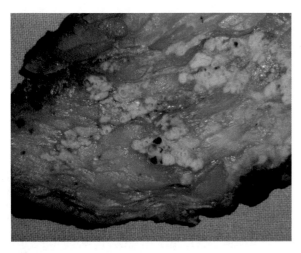

FIGURE 2-18
Gross appearance of DCIS involving a breast quadrant. Comedonecrosis is obvious at this magnification and appears as yellowish or hemorrhagic areas.

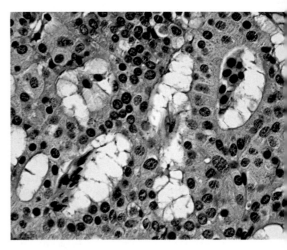

FIGURE 2-19
Low-grade ductal carcinoma in situ (LG-DCIS). Tumor cells are relatively small, monotonous with round to oval nuclei, and evenly distributed around sharply "punched-out" clear spaces.

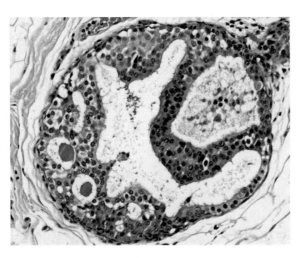

FIGURE 2-20
LG-DCIS showing a more pronounced cribriform pattern.

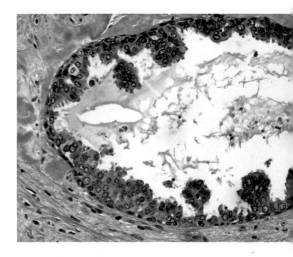

FIGURE 2-21
DCIS showing small papillary projections lined by atypical cells with apical snouts.

Ductal Carcinoma In Situ *(continued)*

■ Central necrosis is not a common feature but may be observed (Figure 2-23).

■ In rare case, DCIS may feature spindle cells (Figure 2-24).

■ Small dystrophic calcifications are often detected in either cribriform or micropapillary DCIS as a consequence of stagnating secretions within the microscopic slit-like and cribriform openings. Foam cells may be found in lumina; however, compared to UDH, they are inconspicuous.

■ At a higher magnification, LG-DCIS features monotonous round, centrally located nuclei with inconspicuous nucleoli and little or no atypia. Cell membranes are easily discernible.

■ LG-DCIS is positive for estrogen and progesterone receptors. It also expresses E-cadherin and low-molecular weight keratins.

■ HG-DCIS (DIN 3 according to the WHO scheme) is an intraepithelial proliferation exhibiting all the cytological distinctive features of malignancy. Central comedonecrosis is constantly present and may be subtotal, with little or no viable cells recognizable.

■ In contrast to LG-DCIS, large atypical cells with pleomorphic nuclei lacking polarity, with prominent nucleoli and a brisk mitotic activity, are commonly documented (Figure 2-25). "Casting" microcalcifications are also often detected microscopically and are often associated with deposits of hematoxylin-avid calcium-phosphate salts.

■ HG-DCIS is most often ER and PR negative.

■ An *intermediate grade* DCIS (DIN 2 in the WHO scheme) is described as an intraductal proliferation bearing equivocal morphologic and likely molecular characteristics that do not allow categorization in the low- or high-grade group. Nuclear pleomorphism is present, but to a lesser extent than in HG-DCIS.

■ *Clinging carcinoma* (FEA or DIN 1a) is discussed in the chapter on columnar lesions of the breast.

■ Myoepithelial cells are present around ducts involved by DCIS and can be demonstrated using antibodies directed against p63 or CD10, heavy chain myosin, or calponin.

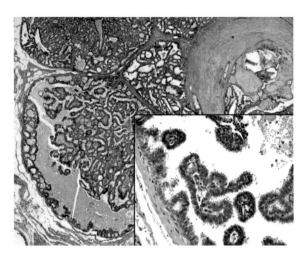

FIGURE 2-22
LG-DCIS with micropapillary pattern. Tumor cells cover delicate fibrovascular cores and are tall to cuboidal (inset).

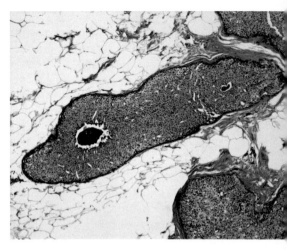

FIGURE 2-23
Solid LG-DCIS. This tubular unit is filled with neoplastic cells showing central necrosis. Slit-like or cribriform spaces are inconspicuous.

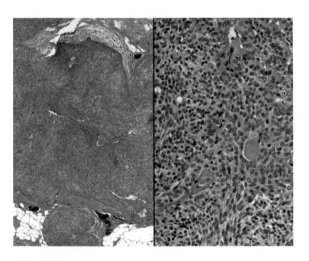

FIGURE 2-24
DCIS featuring spindle cells. These lesions often express neuroendocrine markers.

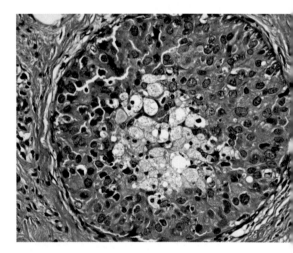

FIGURE 2-25
High-grade ductal carcinoma in situ (HG-DCIS). Tumor cells are larger and exhibit variation in size and shape of atypical nuclei lacking polarity. Incipient regressive changes with foamy cytoplasm and pyknotic nuclei may be recognized.

Lobular Neoplasia

DEFINITION
- The term "lobular neoplasia" is generically employed to define atypical proliferations occurring within the termino-ductular lobular unit, including the so-called atypical lobular hyperplasia (ALH) (or LIN 1, according to the WHO terminology) and lobular carcinoma in situ (LCIS). Lobular neoplasia is often multifocal and bilateral.
- LCIS is further divided into classic form (LIN 2, or type A cells) and pleomorphic variant (LIN 3, or type B).
- Traditionally, lobular neoplasia is considered a marker of increased risk of breast cancer, either ipsi- or contralateral. The risk involves both ductal and lobular types.

CLINICAL FEATURES
- There is a broad consensus for managing classical LCIS and ALH conservatively when the lesions are either detected in tru-cut biopsy or at the resection margin in breast specimens resected for other reasons. In these cases, medical follow-up and/or therapy with tamoxifen are generally considered adequate.
- On the other hand, several authors advice excision or a quadrant biopsy for LCIS showing comedonecrosis or pleomorphic nuclei since these lesions carry a greater risk of harboring an invasive, high-grade lobular carcinoma.

GROSS FEATURES
- Lobular neoplasia is detected microscopically, most often incidentally during medical workup of other breast lesions. It does not possess specific macroscopic features; however, it may be seen in association with other mass-producing lesions such as fibroadenoma.

MICROSCOPIC FEATURES
- In classic LCIS (LIN 2), the acini are distended by small, uniform cells with monotonous round nuclei featuring open chromatin and small nucleoli. Intracytoplasmic mucin vacuoles may be present. The mitotic rate is generally low. A constant microscopic finding is the lack of cellular adhesion and discernible cell membranes (Figures 2-26 to 2-29).
- Comedonecrosis is not an expected finding in classic LCIS.
- Pagetoid spreading of LCIS to the extralobular ducts may be seen and characteristically features tumor cells growing beneath a flattened layer of luminal cells, sometimes in clover leaves configuration.
- Further subcategorization of LCIS is based on deviant architectural and cytologic features such as signet ring cell-rich, solid microacinar, or apocrine LCIS.

(continued)

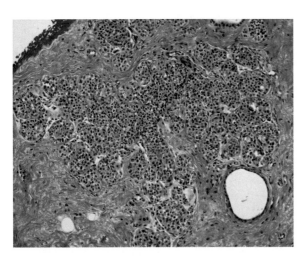

FIGURE 2-26
Lobular carcinoma in situ (LCIS).
Panoramic view showing lobular
distension filled by small to medium-
sized neoplastic cells.

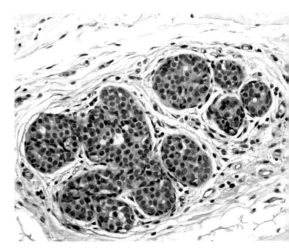

FIGURE 2-27
Higher magnification of classic LCIS.
Tumor cells are relatively monotonous, lacking significant nuclear
pleomorphism, and necrosis or
mitotic activity.

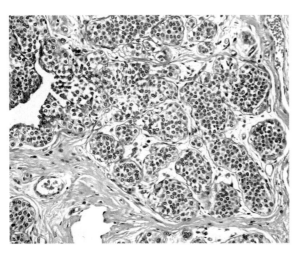

FIGURE 2-28
In this case, there is massive involvement of breast by LCIS. Remarkable
cell dicohesion may be noted.

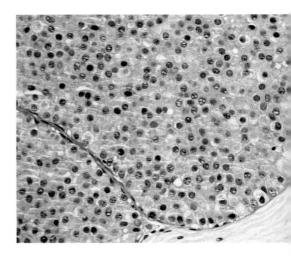

FIGURE 2-29
Massive, solid LCIS. Cells retain
low-grade nuclei and other
features of classic lobular neoplasia.

Lobular Neoplasia (*continued*)

■ Pleomorphic lobular carcinoma in situ (PLCIS) or LIN 3 may be seen alone or in combination with the classic form. PLCIS maintains the same architectural features of lobular neoplasia, yet it shows marked variation in the size and shape of nuclei. Brisk mitotic activity is common and comedonecrosis with associated microcalcifications can be observed (Figures 2-30 and 2-31).

■ LCIS is characteristically positive for high-molecular weight keratins and negative for E-cadherin, that is an immunohistochemical pattern opposite to that seen in DCIS which reacts with antibodies against low, rather that high-molecular weight keratins, and is strongly positive for E-cadherin. E-cadherin is an adhesion protein that is genetically regulated and is lost in lobular neoplasia likely because of a mechanism of transcriptional silencing. It is of value as long as it is useful to distinguish between DCIS and LCIS especially in cases of solid, low-grade acinar proliferation exhibiting equivocal morphologic features. It should, however, be kept in mind that the distinction may be at times very difficult. Furthermore, it is also possible that true combined DCIS and LCIS or indeterminate carcinoma in situ exist. Other important feature of LCIS is its constant expression of estrogen and progesterone receptors.

DIFFERENTIAL DIAGNOSIS

■ Solid microacinar LCIS may be difficult to distinguish from solid LG-DCIS, particularly in cases with lobular cancerization. Ductal neoplasia displays more cell cohesion and nuclear polarization, but less or no intracytoplasmic mucin or pagetoid ductal involvement.

■ Involvement of collagenous spherulosis by LCIS may simulate low-grade cribriform DCIS. The use of E-cadherin may be of value in these cases.

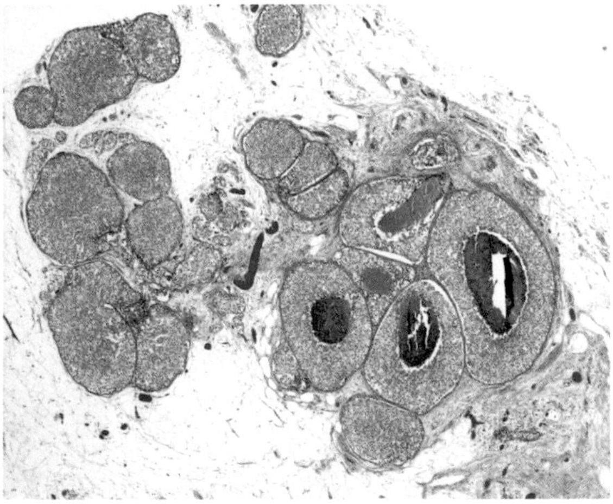

FIGURE 2-30
High-grade LCIS. Comedonecrosis is
evident and may resemble DCIS.

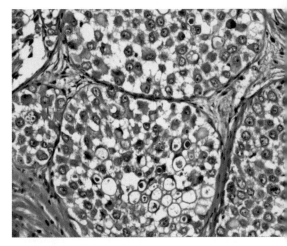

FIGURE 2-31
In this case of pleomorphic
lobular carcinoma in situ, there is
evidence of intracellular mucin
production with focal signet-ring
cell changes. Apocrine qualities
may be recognized.

Papilloma and Papillomatosis

DEFINITION
- Several proliferations of the duct epithelium may acquire a papillomatous pattern. In this chapter, the most important forms of noninvasive papillary lesions will be outlined briefly discussing their salient pathologic features, differential diagnosis, and potential risk for cancer.
- Papilloma of breast is a benign epithelial proliferation featuring a fibrovascular core and variably branching units. It affects large subareolar ducts and is most often a solitary lesion.
- Peripheral papillomas (or microscopic papillomas) refer to multiple, microscopic lesions that can be barely appreciated on gross inspection. Both papilloma and peripheral papillomas are seen in young to adult premenopausal women, although they may appear at any age. The so-called "juvenile papillomatosis" that carries distinct clinical, gross, and microscopic features is not a true papilloma. It is a variant of proliferative fibrocystic changes also known as "Swiss cheese disease."
- Nipple adenoma shall be discussed in a separate chapter.

CLINICAL FEATURES
- Benign papillary lesions are generally seen in young to adult premenopausal women.
- Nipple discharge is the single most common clinical feature of solitary papillomas. A mass lesion may be appreciated on palpation and further discharge or bleeding is sometimes obtained on applying pressure. Peripheral papillomas are, on the other hand, clinically silent. They may be discovered incidentally, in breast specimens removed for other lesions. Some may be associated with mammographic evidence of microcalcification.
- The associated cancer risk of papillary lesions is quite different. There is a substantial agreement that solitary papilloma does not carry an increased risk of cancer, and it is likely that diverging opinions are perhaps reflecting the contradictory and nonuniform terminology adopted for these lesions in the past. Atypical papillomas show focal foci of ADH or DCIS within otherwise benign papillomas. On the other hand, peripheral papillomas are believed to increase the risk of breast carcinoma. It is worth mentioning that the condition named "juvenile papillomatosis" and emphasized before, not a true papilloma, is associated with an increased risk of carcinoma and is often seen in women with family history of breast cancer.

GROSS FEATURES
- The arborizing quality of papilloma may be noted at gross inspection of breast specimen, especially when careful dissection of main ducts is undertaken. Variably sized lesions may be seen and intracystic proliferations are often encountered. Because of stalk torsion, papilloma may undergo partial or total ischemia.
- Larger papillomas have a cauliflower-like appearance and may have a velvety or granular surface depending on the adequacy of vascular supply to the outer proliferating fronds. Necrotic debris may be recognized especially in infarcted lesions. At instances, papillomas are attached to the duct walls by means of larger stalks, have a near-solid pattern, and less arborescent branches. Solitary papillomas may extend along duct branches to a considerable distance. Although a cut-off is difficult to establish, papillomas larger

(continued)

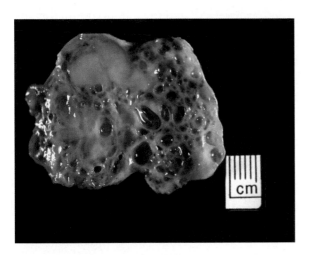

FIGURE 2-32
Gross appearance of "juvenile papillomatosis." Micro- and macrocyst
formation impart to cut section
the characteristic "Swiss cheese"
appearance.

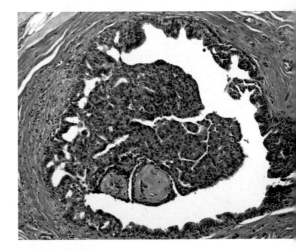

FIGURE 2-33
Intraductal papilloma characteristically featuring an intraluminal lesion
composed of dual cell population.
The stroma is well developed.

Papilloma and Papillomatosis *(continued)*

than 3 cm should be viewed with suspicion since they carry a higher chance of malignant transformation.

■ Multiple papillomas manifest as small, multiple consolidations arising within the peripheral duct system and their papillary aspect is rarely identified on macroscopic examination. A notable exception is "juvenile papillomatosis" (Figure 2-32) that appears as a tumor-like lesion featuring on cut surface, numerous microcystic spaces within a firm, gray-white tissue, hence the appellation "Swiss cheese" disease.

MICROSCOPIC FEATURES

■ By definition, benign papillary lesion of the breast features a dual cell composition, ie, an outer basal myoepithelial layer, and an inner cuboidal to columnar epithelial layer (Figure 2-33). These cells may be easily recognized, although at times cytologic features of either layer may be attenuated due to several mechanical, vascular, or other pathologic changes. The microscopic features of benign papillary lesions (Figure 2-34) contrast with the relative cellular monotony of one cell type that characterizes papillary carcinoma.

■ The epithelium of papilloma, not infrequently, shows metaplastic changes with apocrine metaplasia and clear cell changes being the most commonly encountered types. Another frequently encountered characteristic of papilloma is a well-developed stroma within the fibrovascular stalks that are generally much broader than those encountered in papillary carcinoma. Ischemic or regressive changes are also surrounded by reparative fibrous or sclerotic reactive changes that may lead to entrapment of papillary tissue and pseudoinfiltrative mushroom-like appearance. In these cases, the architectural distortion may be significant. The dual quality of the cells, however, enables distinction from papillary carcinoma.

■ The microscopic features of multiple papillomas are similar to papilloma, ie, two layers of distinct cell types, myoepithelial and luminal. Antibodies to p63 decorate the nuclei of the myoepithelial cells (Figure 2-35). In addition, these lesions are often associated with a spectrum of ductal epithelial proliferation, ranging from UDH, ADH, DCIS, and other benign breast lesions.

■ In "juvenile papillomatosis," apocrine and nonapocrine changes associated with adenosis, sclerosing adenosis, and hyperplasia may be seen (Figure 2-36).

DIFFERENTIAL DIAGNOSIS

■ The recognition of the two cell population is a diagnostic clue to a benign papillary lesion. Nonetheless, cases in which the myoepithelial layer is attenuated may pose significant interpretive problems. Associated proliferative changes of the ductal epithelium further compound the matter, especially in peripheral papillomas.

■ As mentioned above, perilesional sclerosis due to inflammation and/or infarcted papilloma may deceitfully simulate invasive cancer.

■ Stains for myoepithelial cells, including p63, CD10, or actins as well as basal-type keratins such as CK5/6 or CK14, highlight residual basal cells and may be used in difficult cases.

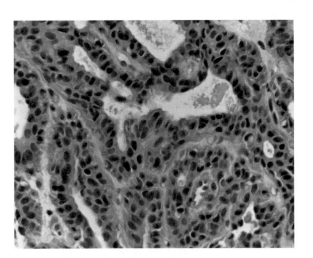

FIGURE 2-34
The luminal (epithelial) and basal (myoepithelial) cells may be clearly recognized. There is no evidence of necrosis or atypia.

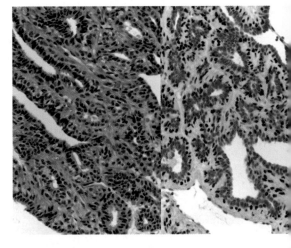

FIGURE 2-35
The dual cell population of papilloma may be highlighted by demonstration of p63-positive myoepithelial cells.

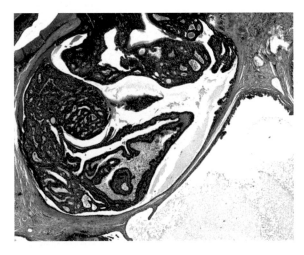

FIGURE 2-36
Juvenile papillomatosis. Cyst with hyperplastic proliferative changes is usually seen.

Nipple Adenoma

DEFINITION
■ A distinct, benign papillary lesion arising within the larger duct system of the nipple that may be associated with proliferative epithelial changes. It often presents with external secretion or incrustation clinically simulating Paget disease (the so-called erosive adenomatosis). Although papillary hyperplasia may be present concomitant with other microscopic patterns, the appellation of "adenoma" should be preferred to "papilloma," since these lesions do not represent true papillomas.

CLINICAL FEATURES
■ Patients with nipple adenoma are generally young adults; however, cases have been reported in postmenopausal women as well as in adolescents. The most important clinical feature, as mentioned above, is nipple discharge that may sometimes be bloody.
■ Paget disease may be reasonably suspected and cannot be excluded clinically.
■ Rare cases of nipple adenoma have been reported in males. Bilaterality is uncommon.

GROSS FEATURES
■ Nipple adenoma presents as an indurated, poorly circumscribed nodular area of the nipple.

MICROSCOPIC FEATURES
■ As in other benign papillary lesions of the breast, a dual cell composition, ie, a basal, myoepithelial layer and a cuboidal to columnar outer layer are encountered.
■ A combination of adenosis (adenosis pattern is most common) and other proliferative changes may be seen resulting in complex microscopic patterns, yet the lesion constantly maintains the typical epithelial and myoepithelial cellularity (Figures 2-37, 2-38, and 2-39). Rarely, squamous metaplastic changes may be seen. Mitotic activity may be present.
■ The intervening stroma may be variably fibrous or sclerotic accounting for the sustained firmness of the lesion. Necrosis and microcalcification are not expected findings in nipple adenomas (Figure 2-40).
■ Often, the proliferating units surround variably dilated spaces. The periphery of the lesion may adopt a pseudoinfiltrative pattern that probably accounts for the recurrences in some inadequately excised lesions.

DIFFERENTIAL DIAGNOSIS
■ Because of the clinical presentation (nipple discharge and incrustation) and disorganized microscopic features, nipple adenomas are considered simulators of carcinoma.
■ The classic biphasic cell population, which may be highlighted with antibodies against myoepithelial cells, is a reliable indicator of benignancy. Infiltrating carcinoma rarely involves the nipple in the absence of a tumor in the subjacent breast proper, and the association of carcinoma and nipple adenoma is only anecdotal.
■ Syringoadenoma and hidroadenoma may be simulated by nipple adenoma, and the distinction may be difficult on microscopic grounds only. However, these conditions are rarely encountered in the breast skin.

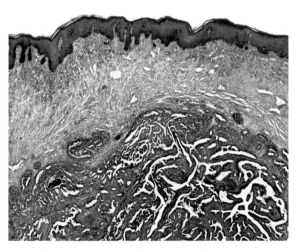

FIGURE 2-37
Nipple adenoma. There is evidence of marked papillomatous changes with irregular clefts and stromal proliferation.

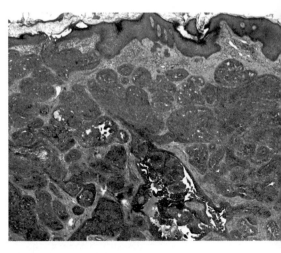

FIGURE 2-38
Nipple adenoma showing more solid changes and focal papilloma formation. Proliferative changes involve collecting ducts beneath the epidermis.

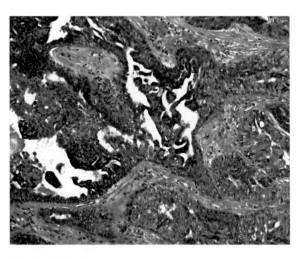

FIGURE 2-39
High-power view of nipple adenoma showing more pronounced, central papillomatous changes comparable to those seen in ductal papillomatosis. Apocrine changes may be recognized. Dual (biphasic) cellular proliferation may be appreciated.

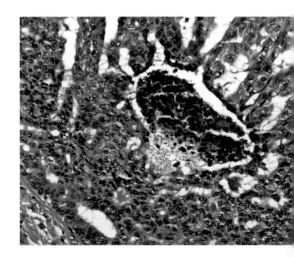

FIGURE 2-40
High-power view of Figure 2-39 showing focal regressive changes with nuclear smudging and incipient necrosis. This should not be considered as an evidence of malignancy.

Complex Sclerosing Lesions/Radial Scar

DEFINITION
- A concerning, though benign lesion characterized by a spectrum of ductal proliferation within a sclerotic stroma.
- With the advent and implementation of cancer screening programs, radial scar (RS) has gained progressive importance especially among radiologists and pathologists.
- Histogenesis is controversial. Due to the peculiar sclerotic changes, it has been suggested that RS is a reactive phenomenon secondary to a previous local injury. More similarities than differences exist between RS and sclerosing adenosis with infiltrating epitheliosis, and some authors claim that the former is a variant of the latter, while others strictly separate these two lesions.
- Although RS has not been proven to be a precursor lesion of cancer, it has been shown that RS is an independent risk factor for breast cancer.

GROSS FEATURES
- RS is a firm, spiculated lesion usually measuring less than 1 cm; however, larger lesions may be observed and called "complex sclerosing lesions."

MICROSCOPIC FEATURES
- At a low power, the lesion has a characteristic sclerosing core with little cellularity (Figure 2-41).
- The inner connective stroma has variable quality, either elastotic or sclerotic to hyaline, and often features entrapped ductal structures with collapsed or distorted profiles suggesting an infiltrating lesion. In an earlier phase, an increased myofibroblastic population may be present (Figure 2-42).
- At the periphery, the fibroelastotic core is surrounded by ductulolobular units that, in classic cases, have a radial arrangement around the central fibrosing/elastotic area, like a "flower-head." A variable spectrum of hyperplastic changes such as usual duct hyperplasia, sclerosing adenosis, intraductal papillary hyperplasia, and columnar and cystic changes may be seen (Figures 2-43 and 2-44).
- Atypical proliferative lesions including LG-DCIS may also be occasionally present; therefore, the diagnostic key feature is the recognition of a double cell layer (luminal and basal cells). Basal cells may be highlighted by special stains for myoepithelial cells such as cytokeratin 5, p63, or CD10. However, in cases characterized by severe lumina distortion, the demonstration of myoepithelial cells can be difficult.
- Multifocal lesions may be present; association with conventional areas of sclerosing adenosis may lend support to views claiming a close parentage between these two conditions.

(continued)

Complex Sclerosing Lesions/Radial Scar

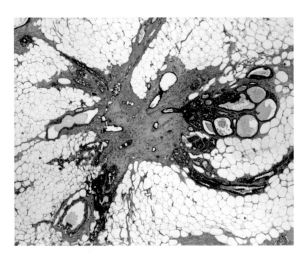

FIGURE 2-41
Radial scar (RS). A central area of
sclerosis is surrounded by disorderly
arranged gland units imparting a
pseudoinfiltrative pattern.

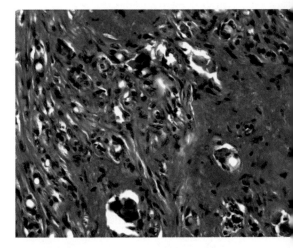

FIGURE 2-42
The entrapped ducts in RS may
have collapsed or distorted profiles.
Microcalcifications are frequent.

Complex Sclerosing Lesions/Radial Scar *(continued)*

CLINICAL FEATURES

■ Because of mammary consolidation secondary to sclerosis, RS may be a palpable lesion especially when measuring more than 1 cm. In addition, the irregular outline secondary to the pseudoinfiltrative, haphazard ductal proliferation may impart a spiculated profile to the mammogram imaging, hence raising further the index of clinical suspicion.

DIFFERENTIAL DIAGNOSIS

■ The main differential diagnosis is with tubular carcinoma. Although criteria have been devised, it should be kept in mind that these are not absolute and that exceptions are more frequent than expected.

■ An overall approach with clinical and radiologic correlation is the recommended standard. In doubtful cases, especially when initially evaluated on core needle biopsy, a conservative excision is probably an appropriate measure.

■ Both RS and tubular carcinoma feature a sclerotic stroma; however, *in contrast* to tubular carcinoma, the following points may be noted about RS

  ■ does not elicit a desmoplastic reaction;
  ■ has recognizable double cell layer in individual gland units;
  ■ the lumina are collapsed and lined by a single layer of cuboidal cells, rather than patent, irregular, most often angulated as generally seen in carcinomas.

■ As already mentioned, identification of myoepithelial cells by means of immunohistochemistry favors RS over tubular carcinoma; however, artifactual attenuation or even absence of myoepithelial cells induced by sclerotic changes is a potential drawback. It should be also kept in mind that focal p63 staining may be seen in some carcinomas.

■ Postsurgical scar may be artifactually secondary to core needle biopsy of Mammotome biopsy and may deceitfully suggest a RS. The latter, however, has a homogeneous scleroelastotic ground substance rather than fibrous connective tissue reflecting tissue repair. RS is usually not marginated by the reactive cellularity, including fibroblasts and chronic inflammatory cells, seen in early scarring process.

Complex Sclerosing Lesions/Radial Scar

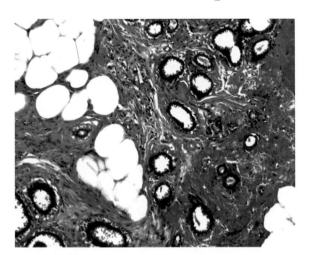

FIGURE 2-43
In RSs, a wide spectrum of proliferative changes may be seen. CCC with apical snouts are seen in this field.

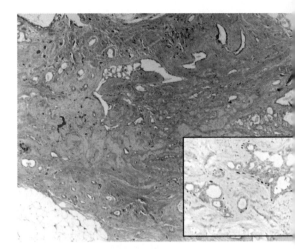

FIGURE 2-44
Hyperplastic ducts in RS. Inset shows immunostaining for myoepithelial cells (p63).

Invasive Carcinomas

3

**USUAL INVASIVE DUCTAL CARCINOMA
(OR INFILTRATING CARCINOMA, NO SPECIAL TYPE, NOS)**

INFILTRATING LOBULAR CARCINOMA

TUBULAR CARCINOMA

MUCINOUS CARCINOMA

MEDULLARY CARCINOMA

METAPLASTIC CARCINOMA

ADENOID CYSTIC CARCINOMA

PAPILLARY CARCINOMA

Usual Invasive Ductal Carcinoma (or Infiltrating Carcinoma, No Special Type, NOS)

DEFINITION
- Infiltrating ductal carcinoma (IDC) accounts for the most prevalent breast malignancy. Since IDC lacks the peculiar pathologic features described in "special type" carcinomas, it may be defined, under a different perspective, ie, cancer of no special type. The special types exhibit different qualities of tumor pattern, cytologic details, ground substance, immunohistochemical reactivity; some of these neoplasms segregate in fairly defined histoprognostic categories.
- IDC has broad medical presentations and variable microscopic phenotypes that reflect the theoretical origin from putative "ductal" luminal cells. As a matter of fact, the designation of "ductal" is probably not fully appropriate, since the majority of these lesions arise from the terminal duct lobular unit (TDLU). It is quite possible that future cytogenetic and molecular studies will stratify this large and heterogeneous group of tumors into more distinctive entities.

CLINICAL FEATURES
- The most common clinical feature of IDC is a palpable lump that may incidentally be discovered by the patient or discovered during medical investigations done for other reasons. The majority of patients are in their fifth to seventh decade; however, a sizable percentage of aggressive cases are seen in younger patients.
- Subclinical lesions are often diagnosed by means of screening mammography.

GROSS FEATURES
- IDC does not have specific macroscopic features. It usually appears as a consolidated mass of variable sizes often with spiculated borders (Figure 3-1). Depending on the proportion of stroma, tumor cells, necrosis, or hemorrhage, the lesions are variably firm. Yet, when a pronounced fibrous or scleroelastotic reaction is elicited by tumor cells, cut sectioning can be gritty. The tumor surface frequently shows a yellow-tan discoloration (Figures 3-2 and 3-3). In a fixed specimen, the tumor area characteristically retracts from the adjacent mammary stroma.
- Multifocality or multicentricity (ie, multiple tumor lesions occurring in the same or different quadrant of the same breast respectively) is not infrequently seen. It has been questioned whether these are true primary tumor foci occurring simultaneously as a result of carcinogenetic effect exerted on a predisposed breast, or whether they reflect disease of a single breast lobule. In the latter case, the multiplicity could be just an artifactual result of the complexity of interwoven and branching breast ducts. This claim is further supported by the close similarity of histologic types, ER/PR expression, and gene profile of tumors occurring simultaneously in the same breast. These findings are also true in ipsilaterally recurrent tumors.

(continued)

Usual Invasive Ductal Carcinoma (or Infiltrating Carcinoma, No Special Type, NOS)

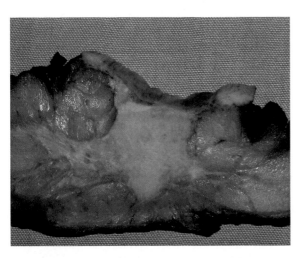

FIGURE 3-1
Gross specimen. Infiltrating carcinoma of the breast invading skin.

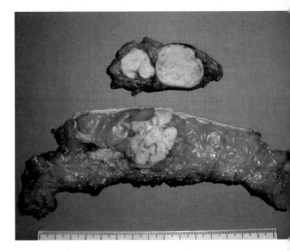

FIGURE 3-2
Gross specimen of infiltrating carcinoma of the breast. *Below*: compared to Figure 3-1, this tumor has pushing rather than infiltrating borders. *Above*: matted metastatic axillary lymph nodes.

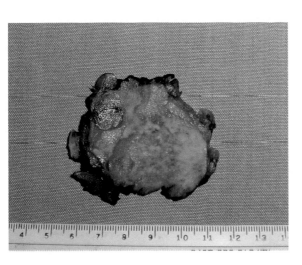

FIGURE 3-3
Gross specimen. Infiltrating carcinoma featuring an ill-defined mass that infiltrates the mammary fat.

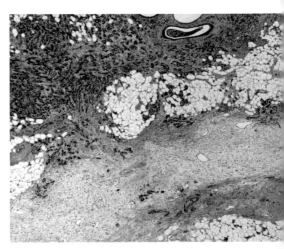

FIGURE 3-4
Infiltrating carcinoma of ductal type. This tumor forms irregular tubules infiltrating the breast fat. Reactive changes and early scar formation due to previous core needle biopsy are obvious.

Usual Invasive Ductal Carcinoma (or Infiltrating Carcinoma, No Special Type, NOS) *(continued)*

MICROSCOPIC FEATURES

■ The tumor architecture is quite variable. In most cases, tumor cells are arranged in discrete tubular or gland-like structures; however, a broad spectrum of morphologic features may be seen within the same neoplasm, including solid nests without lumina formation as well as cords or trabeculae and even cribriform DCIS-like nests (Figures 3-4 and 3-5). Invasion of the adjacent mammary fat is frequently seen (Figure 3-6).

■ Tumor cells are polygonal to cuboidal, have distinctive cytoplasmic membranes and irregular nuclei. The latter can be round and relatively uniform (nuclear grade I) or exhibit a marked variation in size and shape with prominent nucleoli (nuclear grade III) (Figure 3-7) or possess intermediate nuclear characteristics (Figure 3-8). Mitotic activity is also variable.

■ Desmoplastic changes are a frequent feature associated with invasive carcinoma (Figure 3-9).

■ By definition, IDC lacks myoepithelial layer. However, DCIS may spread into sclerosing adenosis (SA) (colonization) imparting to it an appearance of invasive carcinoma; the demonstration of myoepithelial layer is instrumental in such cases. Lack of myoepithelial cells may be confirmed by the absence of immunoreactivity to myoepithelial markers, such as p63 (Figure 3-10), heavy chain myosin, or calponin. This is useful especially in core needle biopsy specimens, when stromal invasion is questionable. However, it should be remembered that some breast cancers of special type may be positive for p63.

■ Tumor architecture (ie, tubular or gland formation), nuclear grade, and mitotic activity are evaluated in order to assign an overall histologic grade within the popular, traditionally three-tiered system, ie, grades I, II, and III (or well, moderate, and poor) known as a Nottingham breast cancer grading system. In this grading system, three separate scores are given for gland formation, nuclear atypia/pleomorphism, and mitotic count. It is still debatable whether these criteria could be applied for grading of infiltrating lobular carcinomas (ILC) and other special type breast cancers.

(continued)

Usual Invasive Ductal Carcinoma (or Infiltrating Carcinoma, No Special Type, NOS)

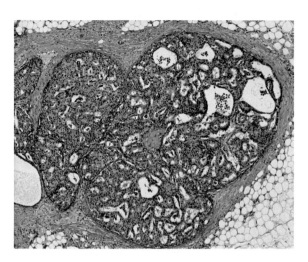

FIGURE 3-5
Infiltrating ductal carcinoma (IDC) with prominent cribriform changes. This is an invasive carcinoma, despite the lack of an infiltrative growth pattern that may be mistaken for an in situ proliferation.

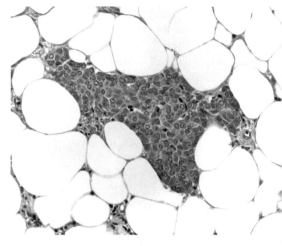

FIGURE 3-6
A focus of invasive carcinoma within adipose tissue.

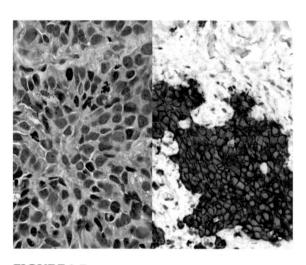

FIGURE 3-7
Poorly differentiated carcinoma. Tumor cells are pleomorphic, with obvious high-grade nuclei, brisk mitotic activity, and atypical mitoses. There is a scant intervening supporting stroma. This tumor also had immunohistochemical evidence of Her2 overexpression (right).

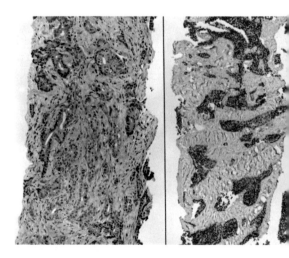

FIGURE 3-8
Infiltrating carcinoma of ductal type, grade II, in a core needle biopsy. There is a moderate amount of desmoplastic stroma. The right photograph shows that virtually all tumor cells are positive for estrogen receptors.

Usual Invasive Ductal Carcinoma (Or Infiltrating Carcinoma, No Special Type, NOS) (*continued*)

■ In situ neoplasm, either DCIS or LCIS may be seen and sometimes it can dominate the microscopic picture (Figure 3-11). The significance of extensive in situ component is unknown.

■ Chronic inflammatory infiltrate may be seen either at the periphery or within the neoplastic proliferation proper. Foci of tumor necrosis may often be recognized. Inflammation may be associated with fibroblastoid activation, increased collagen synthesis, and with elastotic changes especially around preexisting large ducts and vessels.

■ Tumor cell embolization may be seen within lymphatics and veins (Figure 3-12). Lymphovascular invasion assessment should be carried out in areas microscopically far from the main tumor mass. Furthermore, caution should be exerted not to overdiagnose tumor cell nests retracting artifactually from the adjacent stromal tissue which may mimic tumor embolization. Special stains for endothelial cell antigens, such as CD34 or CD31, may be helpful in difficult cases.

■ Perineural invasion may also be seen in IDC.

■ A minor component of "special type" is permissible in IDC.

DIFFERENTIAL DIAGNOSIS

■ Adenosis, either tubular or microglandular, may be difficult to distinguish from IDC, especially on core needle biopsy specimens. The use of myoepithelial antibodies (p63, CD10, and actin) highlights a myoepithelial layer in adenosis and SA; however, their use is of limited value in microglandular adenosis (MGA).

■ Salivary-gland analogues such as myoepithelioma or adenomyoepithelioma may be a source of interpretive problems and their distinction from low-grade IDC may be difficult without resorting to special techniques. Clinicopathologic and radiologic correlations remain essential in all doubtful cases.

Usual Invasive Ductal Carcinoma (Or Infiltrating Carcinoma, No Special Type, NOS)

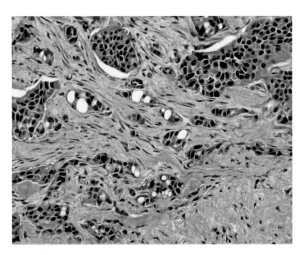

FIGURE 3-9
IDC associated with moderate amount of desmoplastic stromal tissue. Tumor cells are arranged in variably sized solid nests.

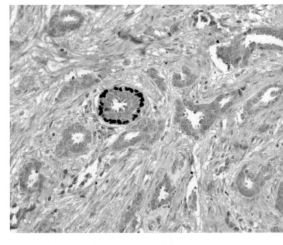

FIGURE 3-10
IDC: p63 antibody decorates the myoepithelial cells of a residual, entrapped normal duct and is nonreactive in the neoplastic glands.

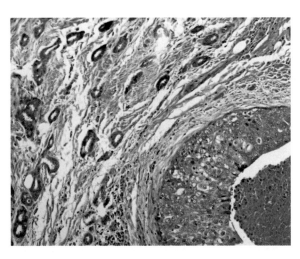

FIGURE 3-11
IDC grade II. A focus of DCIS may be recognized.

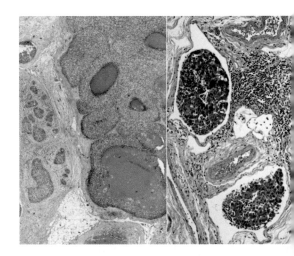

FIGURE 3-12
Invasive breast cancer with prominent necrosis (left) and lymphatic tumor embolization (right).

Infiltrating Lobular Carcinoma

DEFINITION
▪ Compared to IDC, infiltrating lobular carcinoma (ILC) is less frequent and usually affects women in older age segments, although it may occur in young subjects as well. The increased use of hormone replacement therapy has been claimed to explain the increased incidence of ILC in postmenopausal women.
▪ Presentation varies from a palpable, single lump to preclinical lesions discovered by means of mammography or ultrasound scans and composed of multiple, nonconfluent nodules.
▪ Multicentricity or multifocality is often reported. ILC is also associated with a higher incidence of contralateral breast cancer, either IDC or ILC.
▪ Metastatic pattern of ILC differs from that in IDC in that, tumors often metastasize to hollow viscera, internal genital tract, leptomeninges, peritoneum/retroperitoneum, locations that are unusual in metastatic IDC.

CLINICAL FEATURES
▪ Because of its peculiar growth pattern and lack of microcalcifications, ILC may be discovered only once the tumor mass has attained a clinically significant size. Likewise, ILC is sometimes detected incidentally in breast specimens examined for other lesions.
▪ ILC is often not associated with a significant amount of microcalcification, unless it is associated with LIN3 or concomitant benign lesions such as SA. In addition, ILC may not always form a spiculated or dense, suspicious opacity; thus, it may be overlooked on screening mammograms.
▪ Ultrasound scan is more sensitive than mammography in detecting ILC, especially in "nontumor" forming lesions.

GROSS FEATURES
▪ Breast specimens harboring ILC may present with variable appearances. ILC-forming tumor appears as a gray white, homogeneous nodule with irregular borders. In about one-third of cases, however, ILC may present just as a poorly defined, fibrotic consolidation bearing no suspicious macroscopic features.

MICROSCOPIC FEATURES
▪ Classic pattern of ILC features small to medium sized, uniform polygonal cells arranged in fine cords or trabeculae ("linear" growth pattern) associated with a variably fibrous stroma (Figure 3-13). A circumferential distribution of tumor cells around preexisting ducts may impart a targetoid pattern of proliferation (Figure 3-14).
▪ In addition to the "linear" pattern, tumor cells may sometimes show combinations of solid (Figure 3-15) or alveolar/tubular (Figure 3-16) architecture.
▪ ILC is often associated with a variable fibrous or sclerotic reaction. The neoplastic population may be obscured by an excess of fibrous or sclerotic stroma, hence making microscopic interpretation problematic, especially in core needle biopsy specimens (Figure 3-17).

(continued)

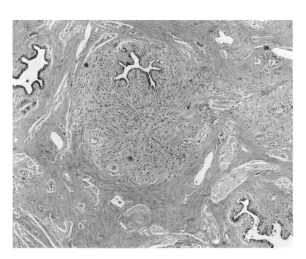

FIGURE 3-13
Classic infiltrating lobular carcinoma showing linear or targetoid arrangement of tumor cells around a preexisting duct.

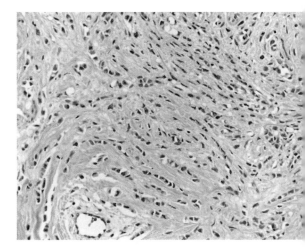

FIGURE 3-14
A high-power view of the same case in Figure 3-13 showing small to medium size cells with a scant amount of cytoplasm. Cytoplasmic vacuolization may be noticed. Nuclei are relatively monotonous, sometimes molding to each other depending on the amount of fibrous reaction.

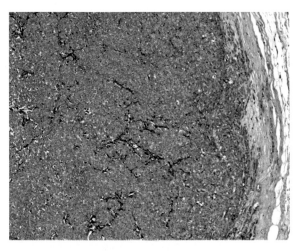

FIGURE 3-15
Infiltrating lobular carcinoma with solid pattern and scant or no intervening fibrous stroma. A pushing rather than an infiltrative border may be recognized at the periphery.

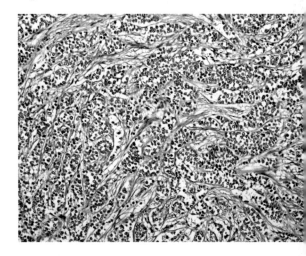

FIGURE 3-16
Infiltrating lobular carcinoma exhibiting a pronounced nesting or "pseudoalveolar" architecture due to thin fibrous septa. Tumor cells are characteristically dishesive and often detached from the supporting stroma.

Infiltrating Lobular Carcinoma *(continued)*

- In several cases, the advancing edge of the tumor may percolate through the mammary fat losing its classic "linear pattern" and deceitfully suggesting panniculitis or fat necrosis.
- A combination of patterns may be encountered in about 20% of cases.
- In classic ILC, tumor cells are small and noncohesive reflecting the lack of the adhesion molecule E-cadherin (Figure 3-18). Nuclei are round to indented with inconspicuous nucleoli and fine chromatin. Mitotic figures are not numerous. The cytoplasm is scant and lightly eosinophilic. At times, it exhibits intracytoplasmic lumina that are empty or filled with mucin, eosinophilic droplets, or vacuoles pushing the nuclei to the periphery and imparting a signet-ring cell appearance. In these cells, histochemical stains for acid mucopolysaccharides are positive.
- Lobular neoplasia, including LIN1-LIN2, is often associated with classic ILC. IDC may be associated with lobular neoplasia as well (Figure 3-19).
- Chronic inflammatory infiltrate is not commonly present; however, cases with a "lymphoepithelioma-like" pattern have occasionally been reported. Perineural and intravascular invasions are not common features of ILC.
- A challenging issue of classic ILC is represented by metastatic presentation in axillary lymph nodes, when early tumor deposits fill the sinusoid spaces without obliteration of the nodal architecture. In these cases, distinction of carcinomatous cells from sinus histiocytes may be challenging due to their low-nuclear grade and discohesiveness.
- Although practically all cases of LCIS lack E-cadherin expression, a proportion of cases of ILC retain it, usually weak and fragmented. In otherwise histologically typical ILC, such an expression should not preclude its diagnosis.
- ILC is very frequently positive for ER and PR. Testing for Her2 is most often negative.
- In contrast to classic forms, the pleomorphic variant of ILC features larger cells with abundant, eosinophilic, or amphophilic cytoplasm often with apocrine qualities, high-nuclear grade and numerous mitoses. It retains a "noncohesive" linear growth pattern (Figures 3-20 and 3-21). Pleomorphic ILC is often associated with high-grade LCIS (or LIN3), and has a lesser content of ER and PR. An increased gain of genetic and epigenetic changes is detected in this variant.

(continued)

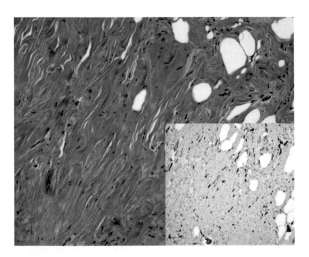

FIGURE 3-17
Prominent sclerotic background in a case of infiltrating lobular carcinoma. Tumor cells are barely recognizable. Keratin immunostaining (inset) was useful, in this case, to highlight neoplastic cells.

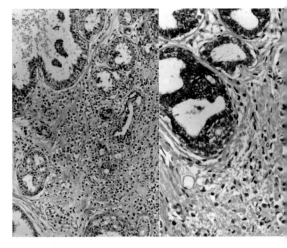

FIGURE 3-18
Infiltrating lobular carcinoma associated with DCIS. In contrast to the intraductal proliferation, lobular carcinoma is negative for E-cadherin (right).

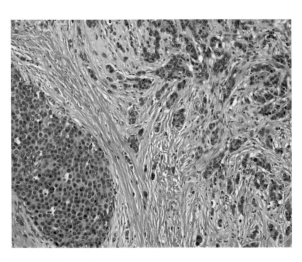

FIGURE 3-19
IDC associated with a focus of LCIS.

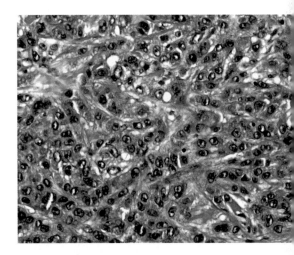

FIGURE 3-20
High-grade infiltrating lobular carcinoma: compared to low-grade lesions, there is more variation in size and shape of tumor cells, increased nuclear atypia, and nucleolar prominency.

Infiltrating Lobular Carcinoma (*continued*)

DIFFERENTIAL DIAGNOSIS

■ The diagnosis of ILC may be challenging, especially in core needle biopsy when focal tumor deposits are present within otherwise unremarkable fibrous or sclerotic stroma. Clinicopathologic correlation is essential in doubtful cases. Step sections are advised in dubious cases. Keratin stains, in selected cases to highlight tumor cells, may aid in difficult cases.

■ ILC growing in tubular or trabecular pattern may simulate IDC. In these cases, the distinction should be based on careful evaluation of tumor architecture and subtle cytologic features. Lack of E-cadherin reaction is a reliable means in favor of ILC.

■ Small cell carcinoma (Figure 3-22) is a rare disease characterized by atypical, cohesive tumor cells similar to those occurring in the lung or skin. These neoplasms may have immunophenotypic evidence of neuroendocrine differentiation and are often ER+. In contrast to ILC, small cell carcinoma features highly atypical nuclei with molding, frequent spotty necrosis, and brisk mitotic activity. Vessel incrustation ("Azzopardi's phenomenon") may also be seen.

■ Lymphoproliferative disorders enter the differential diagnosis of ILC, especially when a solid or alveolar growth pattern is present and clues such as lobular neoplasia are not readily recognized. Clinicopathologic correlations and a panel of immunohistochemical stains including lymphoid markers and keratins are crucial for correct interpretation.

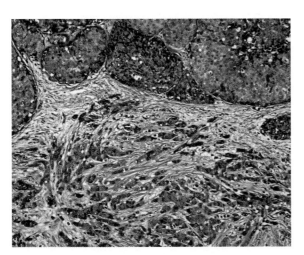

FIGURE 3-21
Pleomorphic infiltrating lobular carcinoma adjacent to a focus of PLCIS.

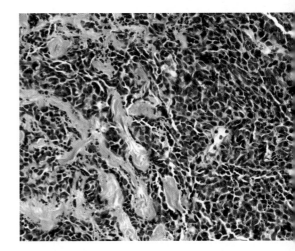

FIGURE 3-22
Small cell carcinoma of the breast. Tumor cells grow in irregular nests with molding and hyperchromatic nuclei. Smudging of chromatin with scattered nuclear debris may be noticed.

Tubular Carcinoma

DEFINITION
- Tubular carcinoma (TC) is by definition a low-grade, infiltrating breast cancer of special type.
- Its frequency varies between 2% and 10% in various series reflecting probably the partial lack of agreement in the criteria adopted for this carcinoma. A stringent threshold of 90% of tubular formation is advised by most authors.

CLINICAL FEATURES
- Compared to conventional IDC, TC occurs in older patients. Pure forms (>90% of tubule formation) have an excellent prognosis and are rarely associated with axillary lymph node metastasis. Skin retraction may be seen in lesions that are more superficially located.
- The overall architecture of TC is such that it is often detected mammographically as a stellate or spiculated opacity. Microcalcifications are very common.

GROSS FEATURES
- The majority of TCs are small lesions, usually smaller than 1 cm, and rarely larger than 1.5 cm.
- TC presents as a firm, curd-like nodule often with a stellate profile. A central elastotic core may impart, to the cut surface, a yellowish discoloration.

MICROSCOPIC FEATURES
- TC has a distinctive microscopic pattern featuring well-formed tubular structures enmeshed in a fibrous or sclerotic stroma. The tubular structures are irregular often with angulated profile and patent lumina (Figures 3-23 and 3-24).
- Low-grade nuclei, of small size with irregular chromatin and inconspicuous nucleoli, either round or oval with their longest axis are oriented parallel to the basement membrane. Mitotic figures are scant. Apical snouts may be present in about half the cases. High-nuclear grade, pleomorphism, and cell stratification are microscopic features that are against a diagnosis of TC.
- The lumina of TC may contain acidic mucosubstances that stain with Alcian Blue.
- In the majority of cases, a low-grade DCIS is present (Figure 3-25), either of cribriform or micropapillary types. In a small, but not negligible, proportion of cases TC may only present focally. Lobular neoplasia may be recognized in combination with TC or in the contralateral breast.

(continued)

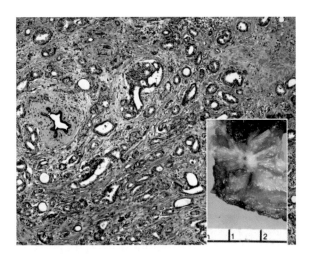

FIGURE 3-23
Tubular carcinoma (TC). This is a relatively small tumor (inset) featuring a low-grade infiltrating glandular proliferation. A cribriform pattern intraductal component may be recognized as well.

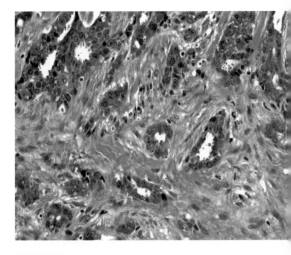

FIGURE 3-24
Small glands evenly scattered within a fibrous stroma in a case of TC. The gland units are irregular, angulated with patent lumina. Apical snouts are present.

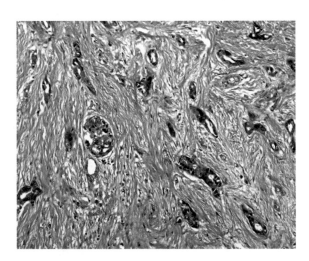

FIGURE 3-25
TC showing a focus of DCIS with microcalcifications.

Tubular Carcinoma (*continued*)

- The stroma is characteristically fibrous and may feature fibroblast-like elements (Figure 3-26). Scleroelastotic changes with scant cellularity may be seen especially in the central portion of the neoplasm.
- A spectrum of columnar cell lesions may be seen in association with TC; Rosen's triad—association of TC, LCIS, and columnar cell lesions are perhaps under recognized.
- Microcalcifications are commonly present.
- TC is nearly always positive for estrogen and progesterone receptors.
- It is important to recognize foci of conventional IDC in association with otherwise TC, since in these cases the prognosis is not as favorable as that of pure TC.

DIFFERENTIAL DIAGNOSIS
- Radial scar (RS) may be a source of irreducible difficulties especially in core needle biopsy. Both TC and RS share similar mammographic and gross features, and histopathologic distinction may prove difficult on a pure morphologic grounds. Myoepithelial cell layer is characteristically present in RS and may be highlighted with p63 or CD10 and other immunostains. However, myoepithelial cells may be attenuated in cases of radial scars with prominent tubular distortion, usually secondary to pronounced fibrosis or elastotic changes.
- Sclerosing adenosis (SA) has an overwhelming lobular architecture and is typically lobulocentric, although the architectural pattern is often difficult to appreciate on core needle biopsies. Tubular units of SA are characteristically much more distorted than in TC. As in RS, a myoepithelial layer can be recognized.
- Microglandular adenosis (MGA) may have a pseudoinfiltrative growth pattern simulating TC. As discussed in a previous chapter, MGA lacks myoepithelial cell layer; hence, special stains are of little use. However, MGA features round to oval rather than the angulated or irregular tubular units of TC, and its lumina are filled with dense, eosinophilic, and PAS-positive material. MGA cells rest on a delicate layer of basement membrane-like material and is not associated with a desmoplastic stroma, as seen in TC. In contrast to MGA, TC is positive for EMA.
- Tubulolobular carcinoma should be distinguished from TC. Although considered a morphologic trait union between TC and ILC, the prognosis of tubulolobular carcinoma is not as favorable as that of TC. Microscopically, it features less angulated tubular units haphazardly admixed with classic ILC, although the stroma can be scleroelastotic. Myxoid changes may be present. Both components are generally positive for E-cadherin.

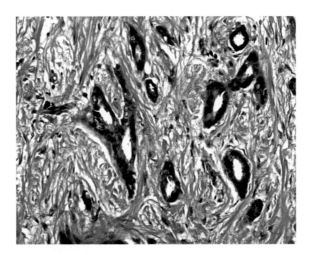

FIGURE 3-26
TC exhibiting a relative monotonous
appearance of tumor cell nuclei.

Mucinous Carcinoma

DEFINITION
■ Mucinous carcinoma (MC) is another infiltrating cancer of special type, characterized by clusters of neoplastic cells floating in a large amount of extracellular mucin.
■ Its frequency varies between 2% and 5% depending on the criteria adopted to define the amount of mucin component. Some authors propose that the amount of mucin component should approach 100% (hypocellular mucinous), since these "pure" lesions carry a much favorable prognosis, in contrast to those hypercellular variants and those with admixture of any IDC component.

CLINICAL FEATURES
■ Compared to conventional IDC, MC occurs more frequently in older patients. However, it may occur in premenopausal patients as well. Mammographically, a lobulated opacity usually devoid of microcalcifications can be recognized. On the other hand, clinical and mammographic appearances are akin to those of IDC in cases of mixed MC, with obvious infiltrating and spiculated borders.
■ The prognosis of MC is considered good. Axillary lymph node metastases are less frequent than ordinary IDC. Yet, mixed forms, ie, MC admixed with conventional IDC, have a greater incidence of nodal metastases than pure MC. Furthermore, tumors with micropapillary pattern are also more frequently associated with nodal metastases.

GROSS FEATURES
■ The majority of MCs are palpable lumps with peripheral lobulation. On a cut surface, MC shows a characteristic lucent surface, depending on the proportion between cells and mucin (Figure 3-27). The mucous substance is dense and sticky.
■ Hemorrhagic qualities are often seen in larger lesions.

MICROSCOPIC FEATURES
■ MC displays different microscopic patterns depending on the proportion of tumor cells, mucin, and stromal tissue, and may be divided into hypocellular (mucinous A) (Figure 3-27) or cellular (mucinous B) (Figures 3-28 and 3-29) variants. The epithelial cells are arranged in cords, nests, or clusters which characteristically float within mucin lakes. Rarely, tubular or papillary structures may be seen.
■ MC may be purely mucinous or it may show a combination of conventional IDC with partial mucinous changes. Recognition of pure lesions is important, since these lesions are associated with a better prognosis, whereas mixed forms have clinical behavior comparable to that of usual IDC.

(continued)

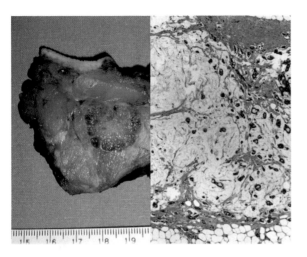

FIGURE 3-27
Gross appearance of mucinous carcinoma (MC). The tumor is well defined and has a glistening translucent cut surface. Classic appearance of hypocellular (type A) tumor with neoplastic cells floating within a pool of mucin material.

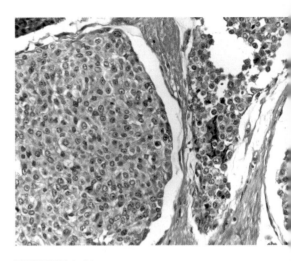

FIGURE 3-28
Type B MC showing a less mucinous background.

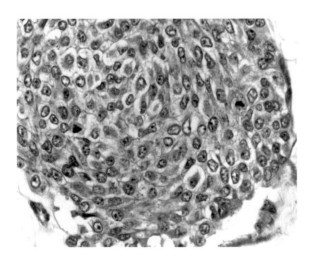

FIGURE 3-29
A high-power view detailing the cell quality of type-B MC, including polygonal cells with moderate nuclear pleomorphism and eosinophilic cytoplasm.

Mucinous Carcinoma (*continued*)

- Tumor cells are of low grade being of small size, with hyperchromatic nuclei. Rarely mitoses or pleomorphic cells are seen. Microcalcifications are uncommon. Intracytoplasmic mucin production is not a usual feature of MC, except for rare cases of MC with a lobular rather than a ductal phenotype and in a proportion of hypercellular variant cases. Micropapillary structures floating in mucin may be seen in approximately 20% of cases of pure MC.
- DCIS may be associated with MC, usually of low-grade micropapillary or cribriform type. Comedonecrosis may be seen in rare cases.
- MC may stain positively for a number of neuroendocrine antigens, especially if the lesion is cellular (mucinous B) (Figure 3-30). A neuroendocrine cell population is detected in a significant proportion of cases, especially in MC affecting elderly women, although their prognostic significance is uncertain and neuroendocrine markers are not commonly investigated in daily practice. It has been claimed that mucinous neuroendocrine carcinoma and neuroendocrine breast carcinoma are two entities in the same spectrum, whereas hypocellular (mucinous A) tumors are a distinct entity.
- The stroma is characteristically fibrous and may feature fibroblast-like elements. Scleroelastotic changes with scant cellularity may be seen especially in the central portion of the neoplasm.
- Microcalcifications are rarely present in MC, but they may be associated with concomitant IDC.
- MC is nearly always positive for estrogen and progesterone receptors and negative for Her2 (Figure 3-31).

DIFFERENTIAL DIAGNOSIS
- A potential source of diagnostic problem is the presence of acellular mucin pool in core needle biopsies. In these cases, step sections are mandatory in order to find diagnostic cancer cells floating within the mucous substance. Ruptured cysts ("mucocele" or other retention cysts analogue to those of salivary gland) may be very difficult to distinguish from MC. A useful clue is the recognition of duct remnants or a discontinued ductal wall with adjacent spilled mucoid material. Extruded mucin may be associated with active inflammation. Strips of hyperplastic epithelial cells may be seen in mucocele-like lesions, thus further compounding interpretive matters, considering also that these lesions may be associated with the full spectrum of proliferative breast diseases including invasive carcinoma.

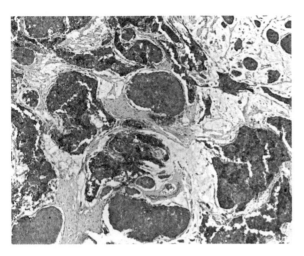

FIGURE 3-30
Tumor cells of MC showing diffuse positivity for synaptophysin.

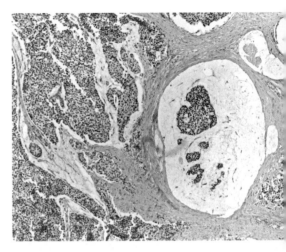

FIGURE 3-31
Virtually all tumor cells are positive for estrogen receptors.

Medullary Carcinoma

DEFINITION
■ Medullary carcinoma is an uncommon and somewhat controversial infiltrating breast cancer of special type.
■ The broad difference reported in tumor incidence (between 2% and 7%) likely reflects different stringency of criteria adopted for diagnosis.

CLINICAL FEATURES
■ Medullary carcinoma affects more frequently women in the premenopausal age and presents as palpable tumor masses with well-defined borders. Mammographic images show a well circumscribed opacity that may simulate a fibroadenoma.
■ Medullary carcinoma has a relatively better outcome when compared to IDC, although it displays a high-tumor grade and it is phenotypically comparable to basal-type tumors. The great variation in patient survival probably reflects the level of stringency, adopted by pathologists, in diagnosing this tumor. Medullary carcinoma with axillary lymph node metastases has, however, a poor outcome.

GROSS FEATURES
■ Medullary carcinoma presents usually as a fleshy, slightly firm consolidation that has well delimited, pushing borders on a cut section (Figure 3-32). Most tumors are within 2 cm in larger size. Spotty foci of necrosis and hemorrhage may sometimes be noted.

MICROSCOPIC FEATURES
■ A sharp demarcation from the surrounding breast tissue is characteristically present.
■ Histologic sections of medullary carcinoma show diffuse proliferation of epithelial cells growing in confluent sheets. A variable, at least 2+, population of admixed lymphoplasmacytic cells is characteristically present along with a minimal amount of ground substance (Figure 3-32).
■ A distinct feature of medullary carcinoma is the arrangement of epithelial cells in broad, anastomosing sheets that may appear as crowded, overlapping high-grade nuclei with inconspicuous cell membranes (Figure 3-33). The appellation "syncytial" is often used to describe this particular growth pattern (Figure 3-34). This growth pattern should encompass >75% of the tumor, although this has not been conceptually accepted by some authors. Nuclei are vesicular, with finely dispersed chromatin, prominent central nuclei, and show frequent mitoses.
■ Coagulative tumor necrosis may be present. Pyknotic nuclei are frequently seen.
■ Tubular or gland-like structure formation is not a feature of medullary carcinoma, although small foci exhibiting a ductal pattern may be acceptable if the bulk of the tumor shows otherwise typical features of medullary carcinoma.

(continued)

Medullary Carcinoma

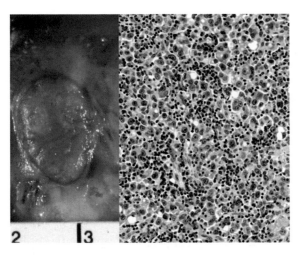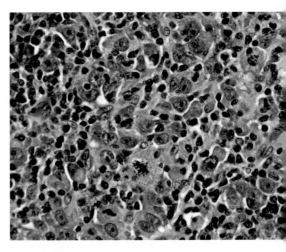

FIGURE 3-32
Characteristic gross appearance of medullary carcinoma showing a well-delimited bulky nodule that bulges on a cut section (left). Distinctive features of medullary carcinoma of breast, including atypical cells admixed with a dense lymphoplasmocytic infiltrate (right).

FIGURE 3-33
High-power magnification shows large pleomorphic cells with vesicular nuclei and prominent nucleoli. Atypical mitoses are also present.

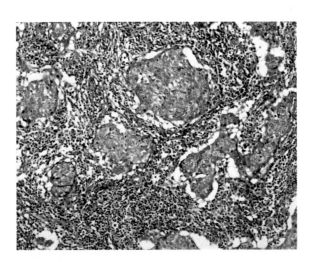

FIGURE 3-34
Tumor cell confluence in sheets often with indistinct cell border may be noted.

Medullary Carcinoma *(continued)*

■ DCIS is not a constant feature, but it may be seen in some cases of medullary carcinoma, especially when attaining a larger size. Changes such as comedonecrosis and microcalcifications may be noticed as well. A lymphoplasmacytic infiltrate may be seen along with the intraductal component. Rarely, squamous metaplastic changes are observed in medullary carcinoma.

■ The inflammatory population may sometimes be overwhelming as to obliterate the neoplastic component; in these cases, the use of keratin stains may help in highlighting tumor cells dispersed within a heavy lymphoid infiltrate. In addition, well-formed germinal centers and epithelioid collections of histiocytes or granulomata may be seen. When a florid inflammatory infiltrate is present, the distinction from a metastatic lymph node may be problematic, especially in lesions obtained from the outer quadrant or the axillary tail.

■ Medullary carcinoma is almost always a "triple negative" breast cancer, ie, it is always negative for ER, PR, and Her2.

■ On molecular grounds, medullary carcinoma appears to be a part of broader basal-like carcinoma spectrum.

DIFFERENTIAL DIAGNOSIS

■ Medullary carcinoma associated with tubular or gland formation, or exhibiting a substantial variation from the diagnostic pattern should be distinguished and probably better categorized as IDC with medullary features (formerly "atypical medullary carcinoma"). This nomenclature is advised when at least 75% syncytia formation is not documented, since below this threshold, the prognosis is not as favorable as with classic medullary carcinoma.

■ Lymphoepithelioma-like carcinoma of the breast has more than one similarity to medullary carcinoma, including frequent presentation in premenopausal age, the "syncytial" growth pattern, and large tumor cells with high-grade nuclei (Figure 3-35). The separation of these two entities suffers from subjectivity and arbitrariness in application of microscopic criteria, although lymphoepithelioma-like carcinoma is most often multinodular and has an invasive, rather than a pushing invasive border. Lymphoepithelioma-like carcinoma of breast, unlike its nasopharyngeal analogue, is reported to be negative for EBV.

■ A heavy lymphoid infiltrate may be seen in conventional IDC, and a distinction of these lesions from medullary carcinoma may be problematic especially in core needle biopsy, where the overall lesion pattern (circumscription vs infiltration) is not easily appreciated and diagnostic criteria fulfillment is equivocal. It is stated that a plasma cell-rich infiltrate is more in keeping with medullary carcinoma; however, especially in the absence of clinical or mammographic information, it is prudent to avoid diagnostic overcommitment and postpone a better characterization, once the whole breast tumor is available for review.

Medullary Carcinoma

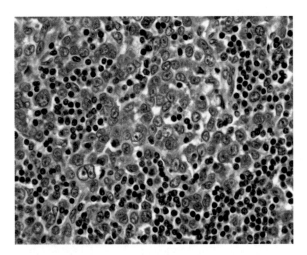

FIGURE 3-35
Lymphoepithelioma-like carcinoma
of the breast. Notice remarkable similarity with medullary carcinoma.

Metaplastic Carcinoma

DEFINITION
- The term "metaplastic carcinoma" (MPC) has been variably, and probably arbitrarily used in the past to define a special type of breast cancer exhibiting poorly differentiated to sarcomatoid features or the "carcinosarcoma" equivalent seen in other organs. The latter is nowadays entertained in the WHO nomenclature under the "mixed epithelial/mesenchymal MPC" heading. In addition to this subtype, the WHO classification includes squamous cell carcinoma, adenocarcinoma with squamous cell metaplasia, adenosquamous carcinoma, and low-grade adenosquamous carcinoma in the MPC group.
- The phenotypic characteristics of MPC have been highlighted by the refinement of surgical pathology techniques and the application of routine immunohistochemistry. MPC is also the subject of important studies focusing on the diverse gene expressions of these lesions.
- It is likely that molecular insights may segregate further this heterogeneous group into better defined entities, perhaps amenable to tailored treatments.

GROSS FEATURES
- Most MPCs show evidence of local aggressiveness, being of large size, widely infiltrating, and often ulcerating the skin. Tumor necrosis is a common feature (Figure 3-36).
- The presence of metaplastic tissue such as cartilage or bone may impart increased consistency or a different aspect to tumor cut surface.

CLINICAL FEATURES
- MPC is an aggressive tumor that affects usually adult women in premenopausal ages. It grows fast and presents with clinically palpable, often large masses. Axillary lymph node metastases are detected in about 15% of cases. Skin ulceration may be present. The low-grade, fibromatosis-like MPC may behave less aggressively.
- Radiologically, MPC usually appears as irregular large breast opacity. Calcifications are not commonly present except in cases with osseous metaplasia.
- The outcome of MPC is usually poor. The best treatment options are yet to be defined.

MICROSCOPIC FEATURES
- MPC features diverse microscopic patterns ranging from purely spindle, to sarcomatoid, to biphasic, or to multiphasic malignancies exhibiting haphazard admixture of ductal and spindle cell carcinomas (Figure 3-37).
- In multiphasic tumors, there may be abrupt transition from clear-cut epithelial ("ductal") areas to sarcomatoid areas, a pattern that still retains the time-honored appellation of "carcinosarcoma" (Figure 3-38). According to current views, the term "carcinosarcoma" should be used only to biphasic or multiphasic tumors showing evidence of heterologous differentiation such as bone (Figure 3-39), cartilage, or rudimentary skeletal muscle formation.

(continued)

Metaplastic Carcinoma

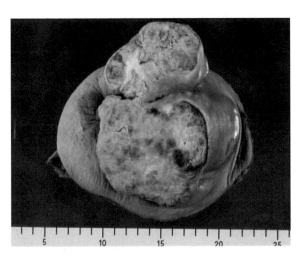

FIGURE 3-36
Gross specimen. A cauliflower-like mass replacing the whole breast and ulcerating the skin in a case of metaplastic carcinoma (MPC).

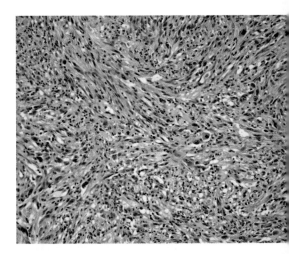

FIGURE 3-37
Sarcomatoid carcinoma featuring atypical spindle cells growing in variably intersecting fascicles.

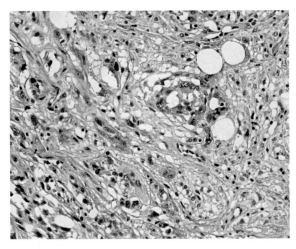

FIGURE 3-38
A focus of rudimentary ductal differentiation may be recognized in this case of sarcomatoid carcinoma.

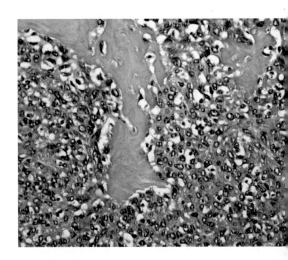

FIGURE 3-39
MPC with an attempt at bone formation.

Metaplastic Carcinoma (*continued*)

- The ground substance may be fibrous or collagen like with desmoplastic features. Chondroid or bony matrix may be recognized in cases associated with cartilaginous and osteoid differentiation, respectively.
- Squamous carcinoma may be recognized in MPC and sometimes it is the predominant or exclusive phenotype (Figure 3-40). Large cell, keratinizing, or nonkeratinizing patterns are part of the spectrum. Squamous carcinoma with pronounced cell discohesion ("acantholytic pattern") may be encountered as well. Careful histologic evaluation and immunohistochemical staining for endothelial cells should be used to differentiate ancantolytic pattern in MPC from angiosarcoma. MPC may also present with features of adenocarcinoma with squamous differentiation, including adenosquamous and mucoepidermoid carcinoma.
- DCIS may rarely be associated with MPC.
- MPC is a high-grade tumor featuring nuclear pleomorphism and a brisk mitotic activity.
- The spindle cell component of MPC is often positive for keratins, usually of low-molecular type in adenocarcinoma with squamous cell metaplasia, and of high-molecular weight in spindle cells in squamous cell MPC. Keratin staining, however, can be only focally positive; thus, a negative staining may not be meaningful; repeated testing on different tissue material may be advised in these cases (Figure 3-41).
- MPC is almost always "triple negative" tumor, ie, it is negative for ER, PR, and Her2 immunostaining. In addition, the sarcomatoid and the squamous component of these tumors are often positive for p63, CD10, and smooth muscle actin suggesting a possible parental relation to myoepithelial cells.

DIFFERENTIAL DIAGNOSIS

- Sarcomatoid lesions arising within a phyllodes tumor may be difficult to separate from MPC, especially when areas featuring the diagnostic fibroepithelial pattern of phyllodes tumors have been obliterated by the sarcomatous proliferation. Diligent gross sampling and search for hints such as ductal differentiation, including DCIS, may be helpful; however, in small tissue or core needle biopsy specimens, the diagnostic difficulty can be irreducible. Positive staining for p63 (or other myoepithelial markers) and keratins may be more in keeping with MPC; however, a negative reaction is not useful.
- Spindle cell carcinoma associated with sclerosing changes may exhibit a low-grade nuclei and may closely simulate a myofibroblastic proliferation such as fibromatosis. These tumors are usually strongly positive for keratins.
- True spindle cell sarcomas of the breast are rare. Specific lines of differentiation may be recognized either phenotypically or by means of immunohistochemistry. In addition to angiosarcoma (discussed ahead in a specific chapter), all the soft tissue sarcoma equivalents may be seen in the breast, including leiomyosarcoma, malignant peripheral nerve sheath tumors, and synovial sarcoma.

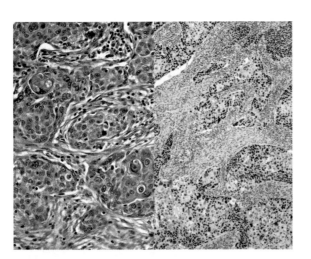

FIGURE 3-40
MPC with epidermoid changes and
attempts at keratinization. Tumor
cells show strong positivity for p63.

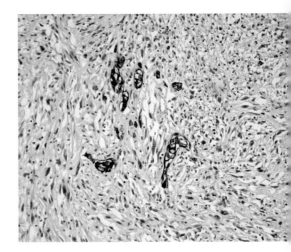

FIGURE 3-41
Tumor cells of MPC may react to
keratin only focally.

Adenoid Cystic Carcinoma

DEFINITION
■ Adenoid cystic carcinoma (ACC) is a rare breast tumor and one of the commoner salivary gland analogues that may arise in the breast. Its estimated incidence is around 0.1%–1.0% based on large series reports. Specific chromosomal translocation of t(6q;9p) has been described in ACC.

CLINICAL FEATURES
■ In contrast to its salivary gland homologue, ACC of breast is a low-grade tumor. A significant proportion of tumors occur in the central/retroareolar region of the breast. ACC of the breast rarely disseminates through the lymphatic or perineural routes. Metastases to the axillary lymph nodes are uncommon; hence, ACC may be treated by means of surgery only. After breast conserving surgery, a high rate of margin positivity is observed followed by local recurrence, sometimes many years after primary surgery.
■ Rarely, lymph node, and even more exceptionally distant metastases of mammary ACC, have been reported.

GROSS FEATURES
■ ACC presents as a circumscribed, lobulated tumor. Most lesions measure between 1 and 3 cm, although larger neoplasms have been occasionally reported (Figure 3-42).
■ Scirrhous-like changes and pseudocystic lesions have been seen in some cases of ACC.

MICROSCOPIC FEATURES
■ The classic pattern of ACC features discrete, fenestrated nests of tumor cells (Figures 3-43 and 3-44). Two types of epithelial elements may be recognized: (a) basal cells with a myoepithelial phenotype lining the periphery and resting on basement membrane-like material. Basal cells have small dark nuclei and scant cytoplasm. Nucleoli may be noted; these cells are positive for high-molecular weight keratins, smooth muscle actin, calponin, p63, and maspin and (b) luminal cells with a relatively more abundant stainable cytoplasm and small central, hyperchromatic, round, or angulated nuclei. Luminal cells are proportionally less represented than basal cells, and react with antibodies against low-molecular weight keratins, CD117, and Cyclin D1.
■ Several growth patterns of ACC of the breast, similar to those in salivary gland ACC exist. The most common patterns are cribriform, tubular trabecular and solid (Figures 3-45 and 3-46). In some cases, one of the patterns prevails, although most commonly each individual case is a mixture of different patterns.

(continued)

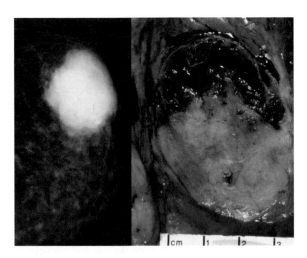

FIGURE 3-42
Adenoid cystic carcinoma (ACC) of breast appearing as a circumscribed opacity. The gross specimen features a tan, fleshy, and well-circumscribed mass.

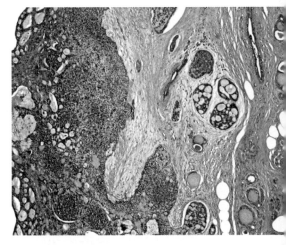

FIGURE 3-43
Solid and cribriform tumor architectures in a case of ACC of the breast. The tumor is relatively well circumscribed (circumscription is not obvious in this micrograph).

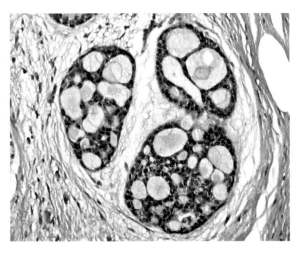

FIGURE 3-44
ACC of the breast featuring punched-out fenestration filled with lightly basophilic mucinous material.

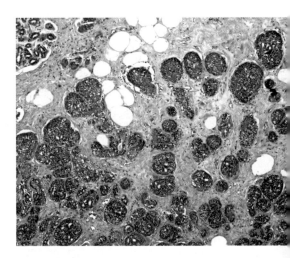

FIGURE 3-45
Solid pattern in a case of ACC featuring basaloid areas with barely discernible lumina.

Adenoid Cystic Carcinoma (*continued*)

- Most of the fenestrations of ACC are punched-out pseudolumina with some variation in size and shape within the nests, and are distended by mucous material that stains with alcian blue, type IV collagen, and laminin. In some cases, this material is hyalinized and eosinophilic. The cells surrounding such pseudolumina are basal type cells. In addition, in much smaller proportion, true ductal structures lined by larger true luminal cells are also present; their lumina are sometimes filled with neutral PAS-positive mucin. The latter ducts may be embedded into tumor nests or lay separated in the surrounding stroma.
- The intervening stroma of ACC is composed of laminin and collagen type IV, often as rims or strips around the tumoral nests or cords. Histochemically, the latter appears as an acidic, alcianophilic substance that may appear myxoid or desmoplastic/hyalinized at the periphery of tumor nests or trabeculae. An artifactual retraction of tumor cells from the surrounding stroma, similar to that observed in cutaneous basal cell carcinoma, is commonly seen in ACC and should not be misinterpreted as evidence of lymphovascular invasion.
- Sebaceous or squamous differentiation of tumor cells may be observed in rare instances.
- Grading according to the proportion of solid pattern has been proposed to be prognostically relevant, although this has not been universally confirmed. A less frequent high-grade counterpart has been described. Distinctive features of this tumor are an increased cell pleomorphism, nuclear crowding and overlapping, and brisk mitotic activity. An irregular architecture of tumor nests or tubules may be noted in ACC, although the dual cell population is maintained. High-grade ACC, in contrast to classic low-grade tumors, may be associated with DCIS.
- Perineurial invasion is not a common feature in ACC of breast.
- ACC is characteristically negative for ER, PR, and Her2 (triple negative tumor).
- ACC may be associated with microglandular adenosis.

DIFFERENTIAL DIAGNOSIS

- Cribriform IDC may simulate ACC, because of its characteristic round to oval fenestrations separated by thin cords of low-grade tumor cells. However, cribriform carcinoma, a tumor related to tubular carcinoma, is composed only of one cell ("luminal") type, and its spaces are devoid of any hyalinized cores or myxoid material. Immunostains for basal/myoepithelial cells are always negative in cribriform IDC. The latter, in addition, is almost always positive for ER and PR.
- Collagenous spherulosis is a benign condition that may simulate ACC, since it is formed by round deposits of basement membrane material surrounded by myoepithelial cells and/or hyperplastic breast epithelium. The separation from ACC may become problematic, especially when the collagen spherules are surrounded by elongated myoepithelial cells. Although the cribriform pattern may be deceitful, collagenous spherulosis is usually documented focally and in the context of proliferating fibrocystic changes.
- Myoepithelial tumors with predominant tubular or tubuloglandular pattern may be difficult to separate from ACC. In fact, it is postulated that ACC may just represent one end of the spectrum of epithelial and myoepithelial proliferation, as the association between ACC and breast adenomyoepithelioma has been reported. Probably, the best criterion to single out ACC is the evidence of local invasion, in contrast to encapsulation or fair circumscription of benign myoepithelioma.

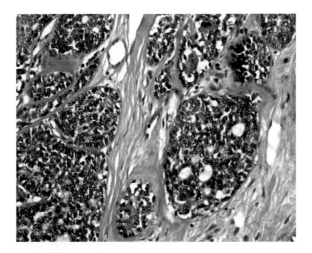

FIGURE 3-46
High-power magnification of
Figure 3-45 detailing focal hyaline
material and minimal cribriform
changes.

Papillary Carcinoma

DEFINITION
■ Papillary carcinoma (PC) of breast is a rare and controversial tumor. Although there is a general consensus on the fact that papillary or neoplastic frond formation is the hallmark finding, there are different views on how some of these lesions should be categorized, especially in regards to the multiplicity of gross and microscopic patterns and their prognostic significance and appropriate management.

CLINICAL FEATURES
■ PC has a greater incidence in adult to elderly women with a peak incidence in the seventh decade. Interestingly, PC is not seen infrequently in males. When the tumor is located in the central portion, nipple discharge is a common presenting sign. Because of the fragile supporting stroma of the neoplastic papillae, bleeding is a common finding.
■ Mammography shows round opacities. Microcalcifications are not frequently seen, when present they are generally of punctate type.
■ Prognosis of PC is generally favorable.

GROSS FEATURES
■ In about two-thirds of cases, PC appears as a well-delimited, soft tumor mass. Macrocysts with intramural nodules may be seen. In a small but significant proportion of cases, it is grossly comparable to a usual invasive breast cancer (Figure 3-47).

MICROSCOPIC FEATURES
■ PC may be divided into "noninvasive" and "invasive." PC that does not invade the stroma is nearly always associated with cyst formation due to duct distention.
■ Fronds of noninvasive PC are relatively long or slender, thin, finely branching, and characteristically fill a dilated duct with surrounding fibrosis. Depending on the plane of section, some tumor branches appear freely floating within the dilated lumina (Figure 3-48). Characteristically, PC has a disorderly growth pattern that is evident at a panoramic view. Blunt or "stubby" fronds may sometimes be noticed. The most distinguishing feature of PC is the presence of fibrovascular cores lined by one type of atypical tumor cells (Figure 3-49). The neoplastic cells are cuboidal to cylindrical, with hyperchromatic, crowded, and often overlapping reminiscent of nuclei seen in low-grade DCIS. There is loss of nuclear polarity. Mitotic figures may be seen. The neoplastic cells may grow in several layers giving the false impression of a "dual cell population"; however, the nuclei have the same qualities throughout (Figure 3-50).
■ The intervening stroma is scant to inconspicuous thus; the bulk of PC is formed by epithelial cells and the supporting connective tissue is just limited to the fibrovascular cores on which the neoplastic cells rest. Sloughing of neoplastic cells either single or in clusters may be noted as well.
■ Trabecular bars or cribriform spaces may be recognized, sometimes resulting from spreading of neoplastic cells on the surface of dilated, preexisting ducts. Microcalcifications are not frequently seen in PC fibrovascular cores.

(continued)

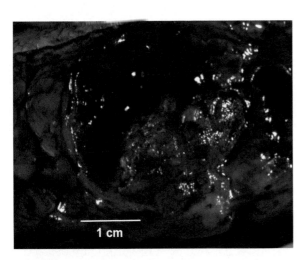

FIGURE 3-47
Gross appearance of papillary carcinoma (PC) growing as a mural nodule within a cystically dilated duct.

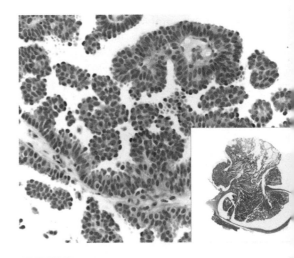

FIGURE 3-48
The characteristic arborescent structures of intracystic PC may be noticed at a panoramic view (inset). Tumor cell fronds may give the impression of "floating" freely within the cystic spaces due to the thin supporting fibrovascular cores and depending on the plane of section.

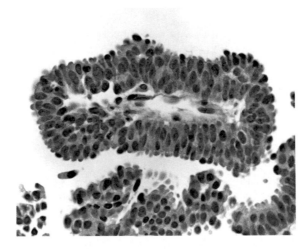

FIGURE 3-49
High-power magnification showing vertically oriented nuclei and a relatively monotonous quality of chromatin texture.

Papillary Carcinoma (*continued*)

■ PC may sometimes feature large clear cells, often resting on the fibrovascular core, mimicking myoepithelial cells, and giving, thus, the false impression of a dual cell population as seen in benign papilloma (so called "dimorphic PC"). An important clue in favor of PC is the nuclear pattern that all cells share, despite the clearing of the cytoplasm (Figure 3-50).

■ When PC invades the adjacent stroma, it becomes comparable to conventional IDC. Invasive PC associated with DCIS is in more than 75% of cases, usually of papillary type. In some cases, invasive component retains a papillary architectural pattern and variations thereof. Other invasive patterns such as tubulopapillary and adenomatoid were also recognized.

■ A distinct microscopic pattern is the so-called "micropapillary carcinoma" in which the tumor forms small clusters or nests detached from the surrounding stroma (Figure 3-51), forming artifactual stromal spaces or within vascular channels (Figure 3-52). Some authors advocate that micropapillary carcinoma carries a worse prognosis, since it is associated with a high rate of lymphovascular invasion, axillary lymph node metastases, and early recurrence. The micropapillary growth pattern may be seen alone, associated with areas of conventional IDC or PC. In the majority of cases, PC is an intracystic tumor. However, stromal invasion may be difficult to assess in tumor-exhibiting pushing margins and in which a rare micropapillary pattern may be encountered.

■ A special rare form of PC is intracystic (encapsulated) PC that is traditionally regarded to be in situ carcinoma. Recent evidence, however, suggests that it is probably invasive as demonstrated by the lack of myoepithelial layer. This is demonstrated by lack of p63 and collagen IV immunoreactions. In spite of this, such tumors have excellent prognosis.

■ Invasive PC is almost always ER/PR-positive and Her2 negative. Tumors with high-grade nuclei and micropapillary pattern may be Her2 positive.

DIFFERENTIAL DIAGNOSIS

■ The distinction between PC and papilloma is in most cases simply applying conventional morphologic criteria, although it can be problematic in core needle biopsies or in tissue sections, where the geometrical characteristics of the lesions are not fully represented. In contrast to PC, papillomas have broad orderly fronds with a fibrous to sclerotic stroma. Except in cases with superimposed epithelial proliferation, papillomas feature characteristically an inverted proportion of stroma to epithelium. Most importantly, papillomas feature two cell types, ie, a basal layer of myoepithelial cells covered by luminar, duct-type cells. In doubtful cases, the use of antibodies against myoepithelial cells may be helpful. The same biphasic cellular features are retained in adenosis-like proliferative changes that may occur in papilloma and impart a deceitfully alarming pattern to an otherwise benign lesion. Other microscopic features seen, more frequently in papillomas, include a more cohesive cell population, paucity of mitotic figures, and stalk, rather than luminal microcalcification. Lesion multiplicity has been reported as a marker of benignancy, yet it does not have an absolute value.

(continued)

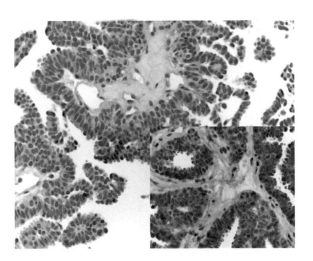

FIGURE 3-50
The fibrovascular cores are lined by epithelial cells, but lack myoepithelial cells (inset—p63 antibody shows absence of nuclear staining).

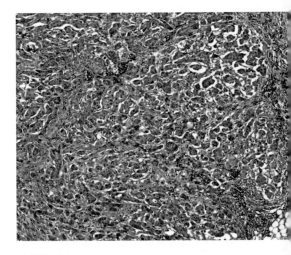

FIGURE 3-51
Micropapillary carcinoma of breast: artifactual retraction of small tumor cell nests is characteristically present.

Papillary Carcinoma (*continued*)

■ PC should be distinguished from ordinary ductal proliferations arising in papilloma, ranging from usual hyperplasia to DCIS. The distinguishing cytoarchitectural features of ductal epithelial proliferation enable differentiation from PC.

■ The assessment of local invasion, in PC, may be problematic, especially in larger intra-cytstic lesions having pushing margins and a fibrous to sclerotic rim of connective tissue. In these cases, the advancing edge of the tumor may have an expansile rather than a destructive growth pattern. In addition, a fibrous tissue at the periphery may be difficult to separate from a desmoplastic reaction, commonly seen with invasive carcinoma.

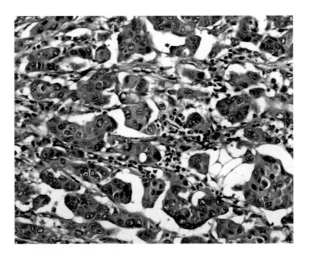

FIGURE 3-52
Higher magnification of micropapillary carcinoma showing moderate
pleomorphism.

Proliferative Stromal and Miscellaneous Mesenchymal Lesions

4

FIBROADENOMA

PHYLLODES TUMOR

PERIDUCTAL STROMAL TUMOR

MYOFIBROBLASTOMA

ANGIOSARCOMA

Fibroadenoma

DEFINITION

■ Fibroadenoma (FA) is a relatively common benign fibroepithelial lesion derived from the epithelial cells and cellular stromal elements of the TDLU.

CLINICAL FEATURES

■ FA is the commonest breast lesion in adolescent women, and it classically presents as a painless, moveable mass. Radiologically, it presents as a roundish opacity. Microcalcifications are not an expected finding of FA but may be present. However, the stroma of old FA may contain coarse calcifications or undergo ossification recognized by mammography. There seems to be a slight prevalence among black women. FAs may also be seen in postmenopausal and older women. On the other hand, they are very rare in males. Not infrequently, FA is incidentally documented in mammary specimens obtained for other reasons including breast cancer. In young women, it may attain conspicuous and often alarming size, with lesions replacing the whole breast.

■ FA with increased fibrosis or hyalinization may be seen more frequently in older, postmenopausal women. Florid FA, however, is not an unexpected finding in postmenopausal women likely due to the widespread use of estrogen replacement therapy.

GROSS FEATURES

■ FA appears as fairly lobulated, firm mass; on a cut surface, it is often firm, bulging, and fasciculated depending on the proportion of epithelial structures and stroma and the quality of the latter. It usually measures less than 3 cm; however, larger tumors are not uncommon. Tiny, slit-like, or microcystic spaces may be grossly noticed and reflect the fibroepithelial tumor pattern. Hemorrhagic changes are not common, although larger lesions may undergo ischemic necrosis or even infarction. An increased amount of mucous ground substance may impart a lucent appearance to the tumor section.

■ Multiplicity and/or bilaterality of FA are not uncommon.

MICROSCOPIC FEATURES

■ FA shows a fair proliferation of mammary fibroblasts along with gland epithelium in a quite variable proportion, although the stroma predominates. Multiple adjacent lobules, separated by nonproliferating interlobular connective tissue, merge to form eventually a visible or palpable mass. Principally, two major microscopic patterns exist, although the distinction is merely of academic importance and carries no prognostic or clinical significance. In addition, both may be seen in the same lesions.

● Intracanalicular FA, in which the proliferation compresses either collapsed or slightly patent duct spaces lined by bland, cuboidal cells of luminal type resting on basal myoepithelial cells. The intracanalicular pattern is due to the artifactual invagination of the proliferating connective tissue within preexisting ducts which on tissue sections may acquire a "stag-horn" profile. When the intracanalicular pattern is very pronounced, the distinction from phyllodes tumor (PT) may be more difficult (Figures 4-1, 4-2, and 4-3).

(continued)

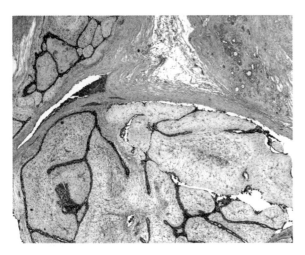

FIGURE 4-1
Intracanalicular fibroadenoma (FA) showing duct compression by proliferating fibroblast-like cells within a myxoid stroma. There is a sharp peripheral circumscription.

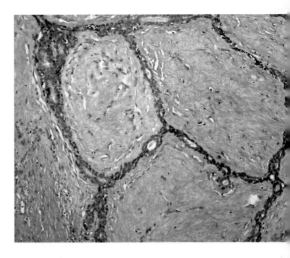

FIGURE 4-2
Intracanalicular FA with more pronounced fibrous changes.

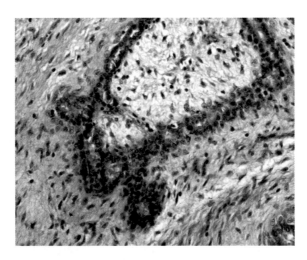

FIGURE 4-3
High magnification detailing the cell components in a case of FA. The ducts are lined by epithelial cells and a dual cell population may be focally recognized.

Fibroadenoma (*continued*)

- Pericanalicular FA is characterized by a radial proliferation of stroma around duct units. A double layer of epithelial and myoepithelial cells is seen in pericanalicular FA as well. Pericanalicular FA is more frequently seen in adolescent or young women (Figures 4-4 and 4-5).

- Regardless of the growth pattern, the proportion of stroma to epithelium tends to remain relatively constant and evenly distributed within the same lesion. Mitotic activity is inconspicuous. Increased cellularity, stromal overgrowth, and more than occasional mitotic figures should raise the possibility of PT (see next section). Lesions with borderline histology have a greater likelihood of recurrence.

- The stroma of FA may be loose, fibrous, sclerotic, or even calcific depending on the age of the lesion. Loose lesions reflect a high content of acid mucopolysaccharides in the ground substance, as they are commonly seen in early lesions. Mature adipose tissue or smooth muscle islands may be sometimes recognized in small amount.

- Giant cells similar to those described in extramammary fibroepithelial lesions (ie, nasal cavity) may be seen in FA (Figure 4-6).

- Infarcted FA may result because of inadequate blood supply to larger lesions causing coagulative necrosis, inflammatory infiltration, and tissue scarring eventually raising the clinical or pathological suspicion of invasive carcinoma.

- Although uncommon, the spectrum of proliferative changes may be seen in FA, including atypical hyperplasia and carcinoma in situ (CIS). The latter changes can be incidentally observed in breast specimens obtained for FA. A retrograde colonization of FA by either LCIS (Figure 4-7) or, less frequently, DCIS may be sometimes observed. FA removed from pregnant or lactating patients show changes comparable to those seen in lactating breast.

- Complex FA may be associated with sclerosing adenosis (SA), apocrine, or papillary changes, or cyst formation. In these cases, there seems to be an increased risk of developing breast cancer.

- The term giant FA is used to indicate lesions with a moderately increased albeit benign cellularity, otherwise comparable to FA attaining a huge size, although there is no consensus on the upper size limit that a FA may reach to be labeled as "giant." Giant FAs usually do not have an intracanalicular growth pattern. Since these tumors occur in adolescent or younger patients, giant FA is often misused as a synonym of "juvenile" FA. In fact, juvenile FAs are larger (or giant) FAs, however, they have distinctive clinical and pathological features, including a fast growing rate sometimes deforming the breast, stretching the overlying skin, and displacing the nipple. In addition, the stroma is more cellular than that of ordinary or giant FA, and epithelial hyperplasia is commonly encountered.

DIFFERENTIAL DIAGNOSIS

- Tubular adenoma or adenofibroma represents a variant of FA in which the epithelial component presents as round to oval units composed of ductal and myoepithelial cells. Lobular units with dilated acini and minimal supporting stroma are typically observed.

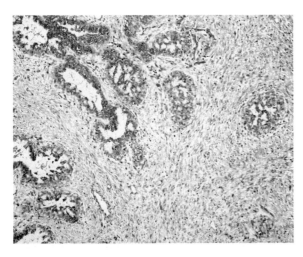

FIGURE 4-4
Juvenile FA: the epithelial component shows evidence of florid hyperplasia whereas the periductal stroma is cellular and myxoid.

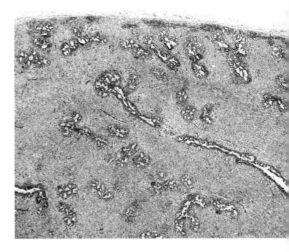

FIGURE 4-5
Juvenile FA showing fair circumscription.

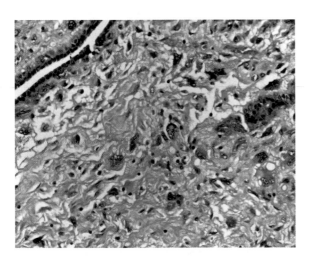

FIGURE 4-6
The stroma of FA may occasionally show large multinucleated cells, sometimes with bizarre cytology.

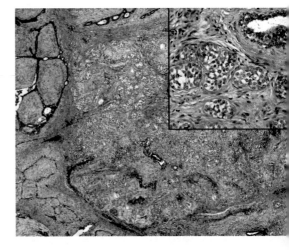

FIGURE 4-7
FA diffusely colonized by LCIS.

Fibroadenoma *(continued)*

- Both FA and PT share a number of architectural and cytologic features, including the intimate association of the stromal and epithelial component. Larger size, gross appearance, and increased stromal cellularity of PT usually allow the distinction; however, the task may be very difficult on core needle biopsy. Excision is recommended in these cases. Certain cases of FA also exist in which the differential diagnosis is difficult due to increased stromal cellularity, and the use of overlapping diagnostic criteria yields equivocal conclusions. In these cases, it is safe to label these lesions as borderline or indefinite "fibroepithelial tumor." The use of proliferative markers such as the Ki67 index may prove of some help. Recently, however, histologic features useful to distinguish the two tumors on needle core biopsy have been proposed—stromal cellularity increased in at least 50% with typical FA, stromal overgrowth (×10 field with no epithelium), fragmentation, and adipose tissue.
- Although rare, malignant transformation of bona fide FA into malignant PT does occur.
- Breast hamartoma may simulate FA by virtue of several clinical, radiological, and even pathological features, including its tumor-like presentation, fair delimitation and rubbery consistency, and stroma and gland proliferation (Figure 4-8). A distinctive finding of hamartoma is the presence of varying amount of fibrous and sometimes prevalent adipose tissue along with complete lobular elements, ie, ducts and acinar structures. In contrast, lobules and islands of mature fat are absent in FA. The stroma of fibrous hamartoma is nonproliferating.
- Pseudoangiomatous stromal hyperplasia (PASH) may occasionally simulate FA, mammographically, grossly, and rarely microscopically.

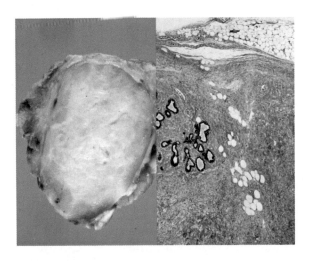

FIGURE 4-8
Breast hamartoma has to be differentiated from FA. Grossly, both
lesions are similar, yet the presence
of mature fat and unevenly scattered
normal gland units are characteristic
of hamartoma.

Phyllodes Tumor

DEFINITION
■ PT is an uncommon fibroepithelial neoplasm likely arising from the periductal stromal cells of the TDLU. Its frequency is estimated to be less than 1% of breast tumors. The term "phyllodes" refers to the leaf-like gross appearance that these neoplasms exhibit. The term "cystosarcoma phylloides," although used till recent times, should be avoided, since only a minor proportion of cases are "sarcomas" and not all of them are "cystic."
■ The relationship between FA and PT is not clear. Some authors have advocated that FA may represent an exaggerated hyperplastic reaction rather than a neoplasm, and perhaps a precursor lesion of PT.
■ Rare cases have been reported in males.

CLINICAL FEATURES
■ PT affects women in the same age group as breast carcinoma patients, with a peak incidence in the fifth to sixth decade, although PT is not unusual before and after those age segments. The more aggressive tumors have been reported in older women. Prevalence of PT based on race is a debated subject; however, Caucasian and Hispanic are apparently affected more than black non-Hispanic women.
■ A multilobulated opacity is recognized on routine mammography and ultrasound scans.
■ PT presents as a unilateral, firm mass. When attaining a huge size, it may stretch the overlying skin; however, infiltration is not seen. Although ipsilateral lymph node enlargement may be noticed in about 20% of cases, this is generally secondary to reactive lymphoid hyperplasia.
■ The clinical behavior of PT is variable ranging from benign, or relatively indolent, to frankly malignant with repeated local recurrences, distant metastases, and tumor-related death. Clinical course often but not always reflects the initial histologic appearance of the tumor as outlined below. Exceptionally, PTs with a "benign" histology behave in an unfavorable fashion, and "malignant" PTs are not associated with recurrence or distant metastases.
■ In addition to histomorphology, an important prognostic factor is size of the lesion. In particular, size may predict the likelihood of distant metastases, while incomplete resection is often associated with a high rate of local recurrence. Complete resection with a wide clear margin is the treatment of choice.

GROSS FEATURES
■ PT presents as a round to oval mass which is fairly well circumscribed and may shell out from the adjacent breast parenchyma (Figure 4-9). The outer surface of the tumor may be smooth, bossellated, and may show vague encapsulation (pseudocapsule). Size is variable, although lesions measuring 3–5 cm are more commonly encountered in routine practice.

(continued)

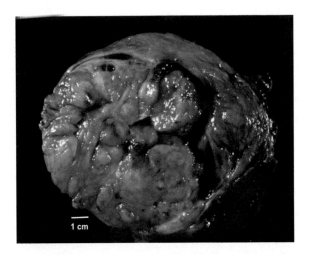

FIGURE 4-9
Phyllodes tumor (PT) showing its
characteristic gross appearance as
a fleshy, circumscribed mass. Leaf-
like pattern may be recognized on
inspection of the cut surfaces.

Phyllodes Tumor *(continued)*

■ On a cut section, larger PTs have a fleshy quality and show a more pronounced leaf-like pattern. Large clefts or cystic cavities may contain serous or hematic material. Regressive changes such as necrosis and hemorrhage may be seen. Smaller tumors, on the other hand, are gray white and more homogeneous and may not have pronounced cystic pattern or clefts.

■ Gross appearance does not enable to differentiate malignant from benign PTs, although the former may have a more fleshy or hemorrhagic cut surface (Figure 4-10).

MICROSCOPIC FEATURES

■ Similar to FA, PT is a fibroepithelial lesion consisting of stromal and glandular elements. However, the stromal component is much more cellular, especially featuring periglandular hypercellularity. In spite of a plethora of studies on PT, there is no distinct boundary between FA and PT, and the degree of stromal hypercellularity to differentiate between the two has never been properly defined. In addition, the issue of fibroepithelial tumors with obvious stromal features of PT, in rare cases frankly malignant, but with pericanalicular growth pattern, ie, without leaf formations, has not been really addressed in the literature.

■ The proportion of stroma and glandular elements as well as the quality of the proliferating stromal cells is important to better segregate PT into prognostic categories. Widely accepted criteria include the stroma/gland ratio, cellularity, cell pleomorphism, and mitotic activity:

● PTs with low cellularity, showing less than 5 mitoses per 10 HPF and mild pleomorphism, usually pursue a more favorable course especially if the tumor has pushing borders and complete excision is carried out (Figures 4-11 and 4-12). It should be pointed out, however, that a small but sizable percentage of PT cases exhibiting a "benign" histomorphology are capable of local recurrence and distant metastases.

● Tumors exhibiting markedly increased cellularity, with stromal overgrowth, an increased mitotic activity (>10/10 HPF), and pleomorphism are expected to behave more aggressively and are categorized as malignant PT (Figure 4-13). Stromal overgrowth may be defined as a preponderant spindle cell proliferation that obliterates the glandular component, as it may be noted at a panoramic magnification (×10). Infiltrating margins represent an additional critical factor. Necrosis and heterologous stromal elements may be considered further adverse microscopic features.

● A third category of PT showing intermediate morphologic features between "benign" and "malignant" is considered borderline, or of uncertain biologic potential (Figures 4-14 and 4-15). The criteria used to rubricate tumors in this category suffer from subjectivity.

(continued)

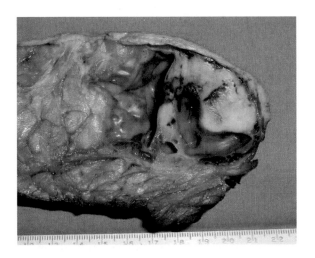

FIGURE 4-10
Gross appearance of malignant PT. The tumor has a fleshy and hemorrhagic appearance and the cut surface is still reminiscent of a leaf-like gross pattern.

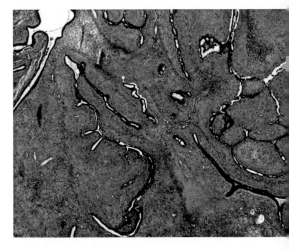

FIGURE 4-11
PT presenting as a leaf-like process.

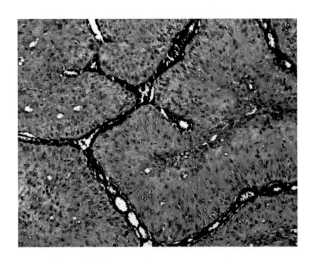

FIGURE 4-12
Increased subepithelial stromal cellularity may be noted. The epithelial cells are cuboidal to flattened.

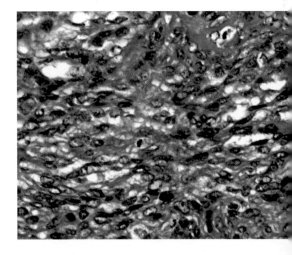

FIGURE 4-13
Malignant PT showing increased cellularity with nuclear atypia and a brisk mitotic activity.

Phyllodes Tumor *(continued)*

■ A special type of PT is the so-called lipophyllodes that is a rare mammary fibroepithelial tumor showing basically all the features of PT with a distinctive fatty component, featuring mature adipocytes and lipoblasts (Figures 4-16 and 4-17). Available evidence suggests that lipophyllodes tumors pursue a benign course.

DIFFERENTIAL DIAGNOSIS

■ Available clinical and pathological criteria allow to reasonably categorize a fibroepithelial lesion either as a FA or PT, yet in doubtful cases, only a diagnosis of "fibroepithelial lesion" may be rendered.

■ Malignant PT with spindle cell overgrowth and/or heterologous elements may be difficult to differentiate from spindle cell carcinoma/meteplastic carcinoma (MPC) on a morphologic basis only, especially if a thorough sampling fails to demonstrate residual foci of conventional, biphasic PT. Microscopically, residual areas of IDC or DCIS are hints of epithelial differentiation. Immunohistochemistry may prove useful, since spindle cell carcinoma type of MPC is generally positive for epithelial markers such as keratins or EMA. Calponin and p63 are also often positive in spindle cell carcinoma.

■ Periductal stromal tumors (PSTs), which are conceptually related to PT, lack true biphasic growth and leaf-like arrangements.

■ Breast sarcomas may not be easily separated from malignant PT, particularly in cases where epithelial component is sparse, because of overwhelming stromal component. In such cases, the best approach is extensive sampling of the tumor.

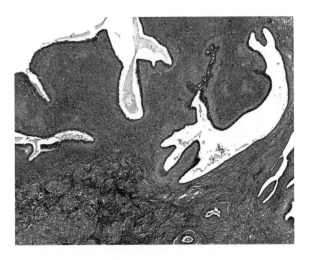

FIGURE 4-14
PT that was considered of borderline
malignancy due to excess of stroma
to epithelial areas.

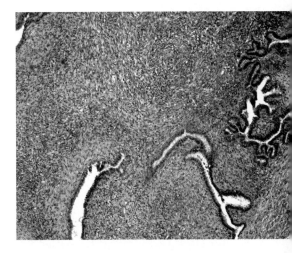

FIGURE 4-15
High magnification in a case of borderline PT showing increased cellularity but no significant cell atypia.

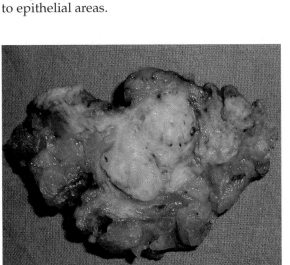

FIGURE 4-16
Gross appearance of lipophyllodes
tumor: the remarkable fatty component of this tumor is evident on a cut
section.

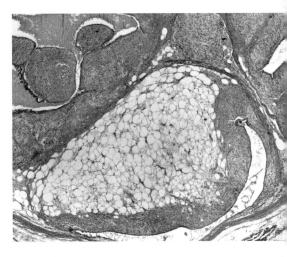

FIGURE 4-17
Lipophyllodes tumor. The stromal
component features mature adipose
tissue admixed with ordinary
fibroblast-like elements.

Periductal Stromal Tumor

DEFINITION
▪ PST is a recently described, rare stromal neoplasm of the mammary gland which is entertained under the fibroepithelial tumor heading by the recent WHO classification.

CLINICAL FEATURES
▪ PST affects women in peri- and post-menopausal ages, often a decade later than phyllodes tumor (PT). A palpable breast lump is the most frequent presenting sign. Radiology shows nonspecific features.
▪ If incompletely excised, PST tends to recur locally. Tumors with a frank sarcomatous appearance pursue a more aggressive course and may cause patient death.

GROSS FEATURES
▪ In contrast to other fibroepithelial lesions, PST presents as a nodular consolidation or mass with poorly defined contours. The average size is generally around 3 cm. A less frequent feature is cyst formation. Fatty tissue is frequently documented.

MICROSCOPIC FEATURES
▪ PST is characterized by a spindle cell proliferation centered around individual, open ducts in a pericanalicular pattern (Figure 4-18). The tumor forms ill-defined, fat infiltrating micronodules that variably merge at the periphery. The glandular units are irregular with outpouching or branching profiles depending on the plane of tissue sections (Figure 4-19).
▪ The ground substance is generally scant or fibrous (Figure 4-20). Myxoid or mucin-like material may occasionally be detected. Necrosis has been reported. Microscopic involvement of resection margins is frequent.
▪ The neoplastic cells of PST are fibroblast-like elements forming cellular cuffs around preexisting ducts. Mitotic activity (>3/10 HPF) is variably present. Nuclear pleomorphism and cytoplasmic vacuoles or lipoblast-like elements may occasionally be observed. In some cases, periductal proliferations may show minimal atypia and paucity or absent mitotic figures. In these cases, the designation of periductal stromal hyperplasia has been used.
▪ The glandular structures often show proliferative changes comparable to those seen in ductal hyperplasia, sometimes with atypical features, or even DCIS.
▪ PST may sometimes progress to, or be associated with PT. Association with other malignancy including angiosarcoma (AS) has also been reported.
▪ Positivities for CD34 and CD117 have been reported with variable frequency in PST.

(*continued*)

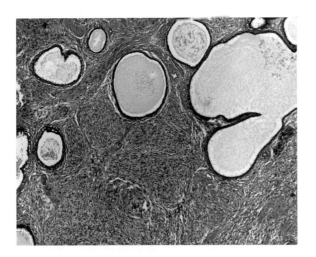

FIGURE 4-18
Periductal stromal tumor (PST) showing a stromal proliferation and ducts with open lumina.

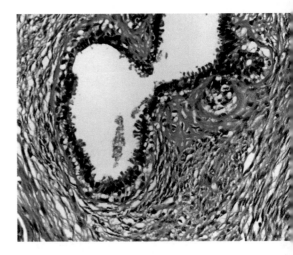

FIGURE 4-19
PST features fascicles of monotonous spindle cells around duct units with mild hyperplastic changes.

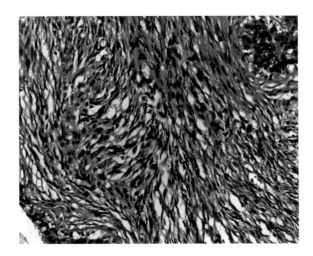

FIGURE 4-20
PST. The proliferating cells have tapered, fibroblast-like features with spindle nuclei. There are rare mitoses.

Periductal Stromal Tumor (*continued*)

DIFFERENTIAL DIAGNOSIS

▪ PST should mainly be differentiated from PT. In contrast to PT, PST lacks important gross features such as the leaf-like pattern and circumscription. It seems that CD117 is more often reported in PST than in other fibroepithelial breast lesions. It appears that the two lesions are closely related, since the development of phyllodes pattern has been observed in recurrent PST.

▪ Further entities to be differentiated include the so-called mammary sarcoma, NOS (Figures 4-21 and 4-22), spindle cell/metaplastic carcinoma (MPC), and myoepithelial carcinoma. The microscopic criteria outlined above enable the differentiation with most of these entities, although in core needle biopsy specimens, the differentiation may be problematic.

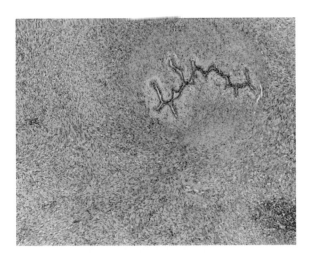

FIGURE 4-21
Breast sarcoma showing a periductal growth pattern around a collapsed unit.

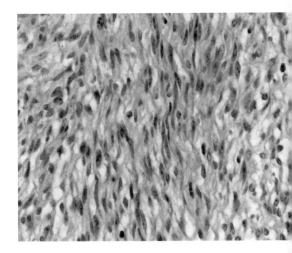

FIGURE 4-22
Breast sarcoma. High-power magnification of Figure 4-21 showing monotonous spindle cells.

Myofibroblastoma

DEFINITION
■ Mammary myofibroblastoma (MFB) is a benign, uncommon mesenchymal stromal tumor probably derived from specialized interlobular myofibroblasts. It is a relatively recently described and well-established entity.

■ A relationship with other stromal lesions of the breast has been claimed including spindle cell/pleomorphic lipoma (losses of 13q and 16q).

CLINICAL FEATURES
■ MFB occurs in both sexes with equal incidence. Adult to elderly patients are affected. It generally presents as a palpable, mobile, and slow growing lump or rarely as an incidental mammographic feature.

■ Mammography shows homogeneous opacities with well circumscribed, lobular margins. Calcifications are absent.

■ MFB pursues a benign course. Simple excision is the treatment of choice. Rare recurrences have been reported.

■ Extramammary MFB may sometimes arise within the "milk line," that is, a virtual, narrow anatomic area that includes the breast and extends from the axilla to the groin, and where supernumerary glands of mammary types may occur as a congenital disorder.

■ Soft tissue analogue, the so-called mammary-type fibroblastoma has also been recognized.

GROSS FEATURES
■ Most MFBs are firm, lobulated masses that measure on average 2 cm and rarely exceed 4 cm in largest dimension. The cut surface is homogeneous, tan, and whorling depending on the amount of collagenized stroma.

MICROSCOPIC FEATURES
■ MFB appears histologically as a well circumscribed, though not encapsulated cellular tumor featuring spindle cells, a variable amount of mature fat, and bands of collagen tissue (Figures 4-23 and 4-24). Hyalinization is a common finding. A hypocellular central area is often observed. Rarely, MFB may have an infiltrating growth pattern. A myxoid background has also been described. The fatty component may at time predominate (so called lipomatous MFB).

■ Tumor cells have bland, bipolar nuclei usually showing a monotonous appearance. Mitotic activity is inconspicuous (Figure 4-25).

■ Further microscopic features include scattered lymphoid and mast cell infiltrates, and hemorrhagic extravasation.

■ Epithelioid, rather than bipolar spindle cells may sometimes predominate, featuring polygonal cells arranged in linear cords or nests.

■ Cases with atypia, increased cellularity, and cell pleomorphism have been reported.

(continued)

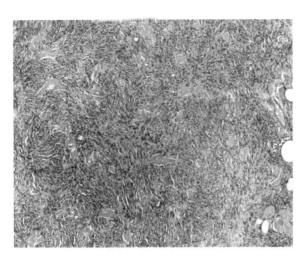

FIGURE 4-23
Myofibroblastoma (MFB). The tumor
is composed of haphazardly arranged
benign spindle cells growing in a
fibrous stroma.

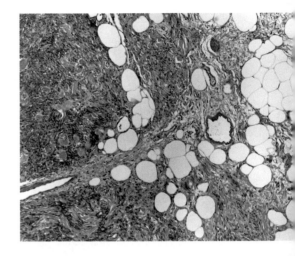

FIGURE 4-24
MFB. In this case, the tumor features
a mature adipose tissue.

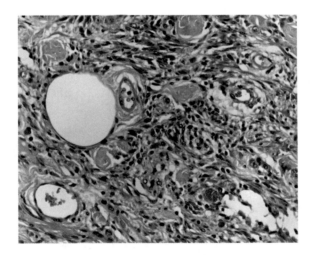

FIGURE 4-25
Cytologic details in a case of MFB
featuring benign spindle cells, adipocytes, and bundles of fibrous stroma
with hyaline quality.

Myofibroblastoma (*continued*)

■ MFB is characteristically positive for vimentin, CD34, ER, PR, smooth muscle actin, and bcl-2. Desmin has also been reported positive. MFB may be positive for androgen receptor. Epithelial markers are negative.

DIFFERENTIAL DIAGNOSIS

■ Several benign proliferations parentally related to the specialized or nonspecialized mammary myofibroblasts enter the differential diagnosis of MFB. For many of them, the distinction is quite subtle inasmuch as they show considerable clinical and morphological overlapping. Furthermore, there is evidence of common molecular and genetic profiles. In fact, it has also been advocated that the mammary fibroblast may modulate through different functional stages, each complemented with a cluster of distinct spindle cell lesions, including MFB, solitary fibrous tumor (SFT), pseudoangiomatous stromal hyperplasia (PASH), and spindle cell lipoma. Yet, the distinction has in most cases an academic importance, since simple excision with clear margin assures cure.

■ SFT rarely occurs in the breast (Figure 4-26). It may be difficult to separate it from MFB due to morphologic overlapping. However, the oval, myoid cells typical of MFB are not observed in SFT. In addition, MFB is consistently positive for muscle antigens, including desmin and actin, and may feature a true myoid differentiation. SFT also is positive for CD34, bcl-2, and CD99.

■ PASH features disorderly slit-like spaces in a collagenized ground substance. Morphologic distinction from MFB may be problematic in cases showing a fascicular arrangement rather than slit-like pattern. Clinically, PASH occurs more frequently in premenopausal women.

■ Nodular fasciitis may occur in the breast area. It may be symptomatic, causing local pain. Similar to its soft tissue homologue, nodular fasciitis is a well-circumscribed nodule featuring haphazardly arranged fibroblast-like cells within a loose ground substance, or so-called tissue culture pattern.

■ Fibromatosis is characterized by infiltrative margins and variably cellular fascicles of spindle cells within a collagenized stroma. Unlike MFB, fibromatosis is negative for desmin and CD34. In this particular context, beta-catenin has been suggested as a useful antibody that is usually positive in fibromatosis, in contrast to most spindle cell lesions including MPC which are generally negative.

■ Epithelioid MFB raises more practically relevant diagnostic issues, since the solid or linear growth pattern of tumor cells may simulate infiltrating lobular carcinoma. The matter may be further compounded by the existence of MFB, displaying an infiltrating and cellular pattern with nuclear atypia, hence simulating more closely a malignant process. A careful overall appearance, including a thorough clinical assessment, is essential to avoid over diagnosis of carcinoma. A diligent analysis may reveal useful hints such as intimate admixture of classic morphology in MFB, including residual fat and spindle, bipolar spindle cells, although epithelioid cells may be at times preponderant and collagenization may be minimal. Epithelioid MFBs have usually more eosinophilic cytoplasm, suggesting myofibroblastic differentiation. Finally, resorting to immunohistochemistry may prove useful, since MFB is negative for keratins and often desmin positive.

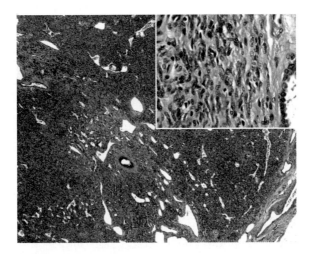

FIGURE 4-26
Solitary fibrous tumor of the breast.
Pattern variegation with focal cellular
areas may be noticed. Vasculature
shows patent vessels with irregular
stag horn-like profile. Fibroblast-
like cells are associated with stromal
collagenization.

Angiosarcoma

DEFINITION
■ Angiosarcoma (AS) is a high-grade malignant tumor showing phenotypic evidence of endothelial differentiation.

CLINICAL FEATURES
■ Breast AS usually arises in chronic lymphedema and in the field of radiation therapy is delivered for carcinoma of breast usually following conservative, rather than radical surgery. The interval between radiation treatment and the development of tumor may be particularly long, averaging about 5–6 years. These patients are nearly always postmenopausal and mostly predominant cutaneous involvement is seen.

■ A small percentage of AS occurs "de novo" in the breast, ie, in patients with no history of radiation for breast cancer. In contrast to the "postradiation angiosarcoma" group, these patients are in premenopausal age; in addition, neoplasms usually involve the breast gland proper rather than the skin and the subcutaneous tissue, although in several cases, the distinction from cutaneous and parenchymal tumors may be difficult.
A palpable mass is often identified. Mammographic findings are nonspecific. In a small but sizable number of cases, the lesions are bilateral.

■ AS is an aggressive tumor. Treatment is often problematic due to the tendency to diffusely infiltrate locally, predisposing to early tumor recurrence within a year of surgical treatment. High-grade tumors are invariably lethal in less than 2 years. Metastases to the lung, liver, skin, and bone are often seen during the course of the disease. Better differentiated tumors pursue a less aggressive course; however, recent evidences suggest that breast AS is most often lethal regardless of tumor grade.

GROSS FEATURES
■ Postradiation AS presents as a poorly delimited reddish or violaceous, often warm induration of the skin (Figure 4-27). On cut sections, tumors may appear variegated and show from hemorrhagic areas resembling hemangiomas (Figure 4-28) to fleshy and necrotic areas. Sometimes, a nodular tumor with ulceration may be the dominant feature.

■ De novo or intraparenchymal AS presents as a relatively large, deeply located tumor. The reported average size is about 5 cm at initial surgery. Macroscopically, it often has a sponge-like or fleshy appearance depending on the degree of vascular differentiation. Necrosis and hemorrhage are commonly seen. Skin involvement is not a feature of de novo AS; however, involvement by continuity may be seen in larger tumors.

(continued)

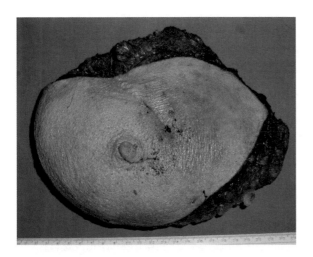

FIGURE 4-27
Gross specimen of postradiation angiosarcoma (AS). The patient had been previously treated with quadrantectomy and radiation therapy. The skin shows purple discolorations with ill-defined borders and a scar.

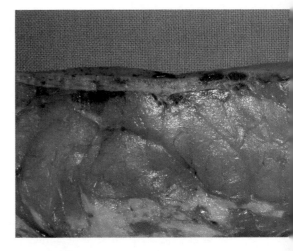

FIGURE 4-28
Gross specimen of postradiation AS. Specimen cut surface showing apparently distinct red areas involving the skin and the subjacent adipose tissue.

Angiosarcoma (*continued*)

MICROSCOPIC FEATURES

▪ AS of the breast does not substantially differ from the homologues occurring in other body sites such as the somatic soft tissue, the scalp, and visceral organs. It may feature the full spectrum of endothelial proliferation, from the well-differentiated forms showing the classic "freely anastomosing vascular channels" to poorly differentiated, pleomorphic neoplasms with barely discernible evidence of vascular differentiation (Figure 4-29). Well-differentiated ASs often have a deceitful low-grade appearance with an orderly, empty space pattern, scant mitoses, and paucity of mitotic figures (Figure 4-30), although there is evidence of diffuse infiltration of breast tissue and stromal dissection. Often, there is microscopic involvement of the resection margins. Poorly differentiated tumors, on the other hand, display solid or predominantly spindle cell areas, and are frequently highly necrotic and hemorrhagic.

▪ Well and poorly differentiated tumors have a comparable incidence; less frequently, breast AS may feature an intermediate degree of differentiation with vasoformative elements and distinctive papillary projections within lumina, cell multilayering, and scattered mitoses. There is also a cytologic evidence of endothelial differentiation such as well-developed intracytoplasmic spaces containing blood cells or optically clear, rudimentary vacuoles. Well and poorly differentiated areas may coexist in the same neoplasm.

▪ In a small but sizable percentage of cases, AS may show a predominance of epithelioid cells with little evidence of endothelial differentiation (Figures 4-31 and 4-32).

▪ Postradiation AS is associated, and often preceded by abnormal, nonneoplastic vascular changes especially in the superficial and mid-dermis. These atypical vascular lesions feature irregular, patent spaces enmeshed in a fibrous to sclerotic stroma, and a freely anastomosing vascular pattern may be recognized. Significant cellular atypia is lacking; however, the endothelial cells lining the spaces show hobnailing hyperchromatic nuclei (Figure 4-33). Inflammatory cells are commonly present.

▪ Similar to their extramammary counterpart, breast AS is immunohistochemically positive for factor VIII-related antigen, CD31, CD34, and Fli-1. None of these antigens are totally specific for diagnostic confirmation; however, when used in panels against other antigens, CD31 is probably the best marker for endothelial differentiation. It should be remembered that epithelioid AS may show some aberrant positivity for cytokeratins, CD30, or S100; thus, the interpretation of immunohistochemical (IHC) stains should be always carried out in light of the proper clinical and pathological context of each case.

DIFFERENTIAL DIAGNOSIS

▪ The better differentiated forms of AS may show deceitfully bland features potentially simulating a benign vascular tumor such as capillary hemangioma or angiolipoma. These features are seen especially at the periphery of the tumor. The diagnostic difficulty in these cases is further compounded in core needle biopsy or in small specimens. Evaluation of the entire lesion or re-biopsy is generally advisable in large and clinically suspicious tumors.

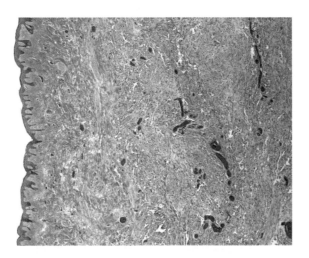

FIGURE 4-29
AS. The anastomosing vascular channels of this tumor may be noticed at a panoramic view. Peripheral dissection of the dermal collagen by the neoplastic cells is also evident.

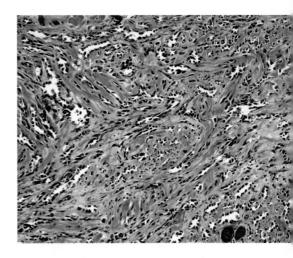

FIGURE 4-30
AS. The proliferation is composed of spindle to epithelioid cells with hyperchromatic nuclei.

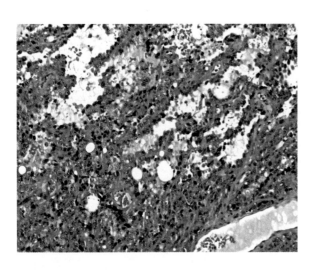

FIGURE 4-31
Epithelioid AS. Tumor cells have a remarkable resemblance to any other epitheloid tumor, although the vascular arrangement is evident.

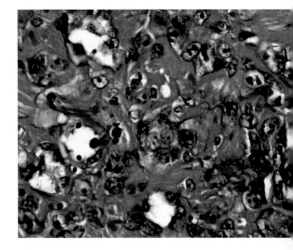

FIGURE 4-32
Epithelioid AS. Rudimentary endothelial differentiation may be noticed with intracytoplasmic vacuoles filled with red blood cells.

Angiosarcoma (*continued*)

- Epithelioid hemangioendothelioma of soft tissue may extensively involve the breast gland (Figure 4-34). Tumor cells feature low-grade nuclei and attempt at endothelial differentiation (Figure 4-35).

- Poorly differentiated squamous carcinoma exhibiting an acantholytic pattern has been rarely described in the breast. Similar to its homologue in mucosal sites of the upper aerodigestive tract, these tumors may deceitfully mimic a vascular neoplasm, in particular the freely anastomosing vascular pattern of AS. However, acantholytic carcinoma usually exhibits features of squamous differentiation in other foci of the tumor and the degree of cell atypia, mitotic activity, and pleomorphism is much more pronounced than is seen in well differentiated AS. Immunohistochemically, acantholytic carcinoma is positive for keratin and negative for endothelial markers, whereas an inverse profile is expected in AS.

- Poorly differentiated AS presenting as solid or high-grade spindle cell proliferations are difficult to be recognized microscopically, unless there is a focal evidence of endothelial differentiation. These tumors may simulate a broad spectrum of malignancies, from spindle cell MPC (see page 88 on Metaplastic Carcinoma) to other, nonvascular breast sarcomas. The latter group represents heterogeneous group of entities occurring in the soft tissue and are quite rare compared to spindle cell carcinoma and AS. Care must be exercised before making a diagnosis of breast sarcoma, especially in limited tissue samples.

- Kaposi sarcoma (KS) may be considered in the differential diagnosis of AS. Cutaneous lesions of KS do not differ from the plaque, erythematous, or nodular lesions seen in sporadic or epidemic forms encountered in other skin locations. Yet, they do not occur in the setting of previous radiation therapy; KS presenting as a solitary breast tumor is quite uncommon, and most if not all of mammary lesions are detected in immunocompromised hosts with systemic KS and clinical evidence of HIV infection. In addition to clinical criteria, KS shows proliferation of bland spindle cells within a variably sclerotic stroma that may show hemosiderin incrustation. Slit-like spaces are often filled with erythrocytes and/or hyaline bodies. CD34 and especially HHV8 antibodies are useful to support the diagnosis of KS in doubtful cases.

- Among nonneoplastic conditions, finally, pseudoangiomatous hyperplasia may enter the differential diagnosis of AS, especially in cases featuring cellular fascicles. Lack of atypia, bland cellularity, and negativity for vascular markers aid in the diagnosis.

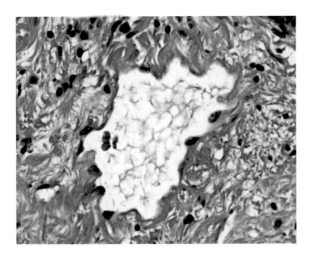

FIGURE 4-33
Atypical postradiation changes in
a dermal vessel of breast showing
irregularly dilated lumen and hyperchromatic cells.

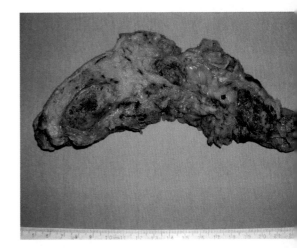

FIGURE 4-34
Gross specimen of epithelioid hemangioendothelioma of the breast: multiple spongy to flesh-like nodules may
be recognized (courtesy of
Dr Tiziana Salviato, Pordenone
Hospital, Italy).

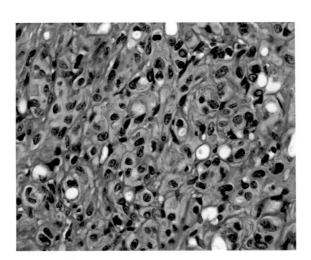

FIGURE 4-35
Epithelioid hemangioendothelioma:
the tumors have low-grade features
along with microscopic evidence of
endothelial differentiation.

Metastatic Tumors to the Breast

5

MELANOMA

MISCELLANEA—OTHER METASTATIC TUMORS

LYMPHOMA AND HEMATOPOIETIC DISORDERS

Melanoma

DEFINITION

■ Malignant melanoma arising primarily in the breast is exceedingly rare and, unless disproven by clinical evidence, it has to be considered metastatic mostly from a primary cutaneous lesion.

■ This problem may be somehow encountered in consultation practice when slides from a "poorly differentiated breast cancer" are submitted to a referral center laboratory for the evaluation of hormone receptors or Her2 status.

CLINICAL FEATURES

■ Breasts may be involved in cases of widespread metastatic malignant melanoma (MMM), with either cutaneous or parenchymal primaries. Clinical history may reveal a primary skin tumor biopsied many years prior, or it may be a metastasis from a regressed primary tumor.

GROSS FEATURES

■ MMM nodules appear as fleshy consolidations reflecting their high cell to stroma ratio. Pigmented tumors are notably brownish, yet nonpigmented tumors are often seen. Lesions are well defined rather than infiltrating.

MICROSCOPIC FEATURES

■ It is well known that MMMs may exhibit an extraordinary phenotypic variability and their microscopic interpretation at metastatic sites may be problematic.

■ Most MMMs grow in sheets of polygonal or spindle malignant cells. Useful diagnostic hints that may raise the index of suspicion of melanoma include cell discohesiveness and abundant, large prominent nucleoli, stainable or glassy cytoplasm. Pigment may be present, usually dust-like type but it may be totally absent (Figures 5-1 and 5-2).

■ MMM is commonly positive for S100 protein, and a strong nuclear and cytoplasmic staining is expected in the majority of cases. The more specific melanoma markers such as HMB45 and Melan A may also be positive; however, a negative staining does not preclude a diagnosis of melanoma in the proper context. Keratins are usually, but not always negative. ER, PR, and Her2 are negative.

(continued)

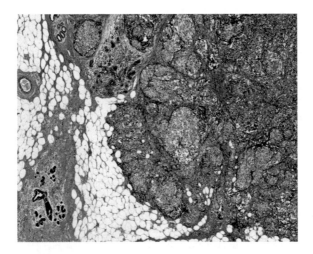

FIGURE 5-1
Metastatic melanoma. The tumor
features nests of atypical epithelioid
to spindle cells. Some foci grow along
the preexistent duct units.

Melanoma *(continued)*

DIFFERENTIAL DIAGNOSIS

- Despite the protean tumor appearances including variable shape and size of tumor cells, changing qualities of the ground substance, etc., the diagnosis of MMM to the breast is relatively easy to make, especially if there is a history of melanoma and/or the patient has evidence of multiple or systemic metastases.

- However, clinical evidence may sometimes be missing or not informative, as for example in cases with remote cutaneous biopsy lesions, even neglected by the patient, or when primary melanoma has regressed or is located in extracutaneous or visceral sites.

- Microscopic interpretation may also be problematic in cases of epithelioid MMM presenting as a single breast tumor, hence simulating clinically and histologically a primary malignancy. Hints raising the index of suspicion are the discohesive growth pattern that most melanomas have, the relatively abundant, stainable, or glassy quality of cytoplasm imparting a rhabdoid cell morphology, and vesicular nuclei with prominent nucleoli or nuclei with cytoplasmic inclusions. Intracellular melanin is a feature suggesting melanoma, yet rare, anecdotal cases of breast carcinoma producing melanin (or "melanotic carcinoma") and coexistent breast carcinoma and MMM have been reported.

- Immunohistochemistry may be applied to recognize MMM. However, it should be kept in mind that MMM may be at times completely negative for melanoma markers and S100 protein. Furthermore, HMB45 immunoreactivity has rarely been documented in breast cancer and in normal breast tissue.

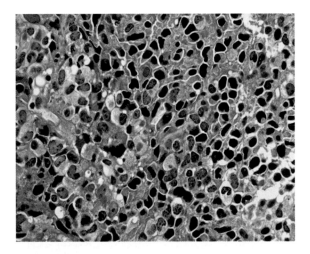

FIGURE 5-2
Metastatic melanoma. This tumor
is composed of highly atypical
malignant cells showing nuclear
pleomorphism and lack cohesiveness.
Distinction from primary carcinoma
may be difficult on a pure morphologic basis.

Miscellanea—Other Metastatic Tumors

DEFINITION

▪ Breast is not uncommon site of metastatic tumors. Their clinical relevance is important, especially in patients with remote history of primary tumors elsewhere, or no history at all. In addition to melanoma and hematopoietic disorders, which have been addressed separately, several tumors have been described.

▪ Although anecdotal examples of many different histologic types have been reported, either epithelial or mesenchymal, a fair subset of tumors is more frequently observed. Whether this merely reflects a chance phenomenon or might result from local factors creating a favoring milieu for metastatic implant and growth is largely speculative.

▪ It is therefore important not to preclude the possibility of a metastatic tumor to the breast, when dealing with tumor displaying unusual clinical manifestations.

CLINICAL FEATURES

▪ Most metastases to the breast are seen in patients who have already clinical evidence of systemic metastatic disease. A small fraction of breast metastases may be seen in males affected by gynecomastia, either due to medical treatments or chromosomal aberration (Klinefelter's disease).

▪ Presentation may vary, from single to multiple or rarely bilateral tumors. A predilection for the outer quadrants has been reported. Mammography reveals gland opacity usually devoid of microcalcifications and lacking the spiculated profile of usual invasive carcinoma. Important exceptions are ovarian serous carcinoma, and papillary thyroid carcinoma, which not infrequently metastasize to the breast.

▪ The clinical incidence of metastases to the breast is low but probably underestimated, since a number of autopsy studies indicate that most lesions are often not recognized clinically.

GROSS FEATURES

▪ Metastases to the breast are firm and well circumscribed. Other qualities such as necrosis or hemorrhage depend on the characteristic features of the primary tumor.

MICROSCOPIC FEATURES

▪ The histopathologic appearance of metastases to the breast is usually similar to that of the primary tumor (Figures 5-3, 5-4, 5-5, 5-6, and 5-7). Frequent albeit nonspecific findings include circumscription and vascular invasion.

▪ Larger studies show a relative prevalence of ovarian, lung, gastric, and renal carcinoma as the most commonly metastasizing neoplasms. Anecdotal examples of most malignant tumors may be retrieved from the medical literature.

(continued)

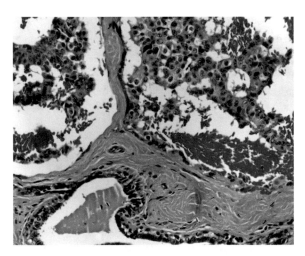

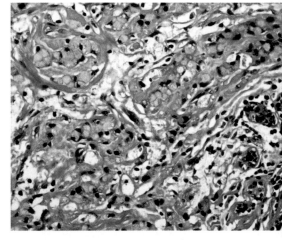

FIGURE 5-3
Metastatic pulmonary neuroendocrine carcinoma. Tumor cells grow in trabecular arrangement and are composed of small epithelial cells with round to oval nuclei.

FIGURE 5-4
Metastatic signet-ring cell carcinoma of the stomach. Note the unremarkable adjacent lobule.

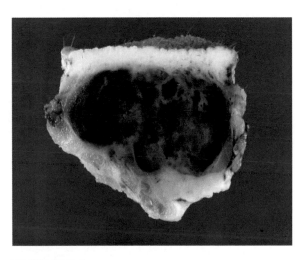

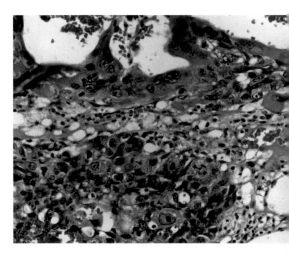

FIGURE 5-5
Gross specimen. Metastatic choriocarcinoma to the breast manifesting as a spongy, hemorrhagic mass with ill-defined borders. The patient had a history of pregnancy 8 years before.

FIGURE 5-6
Metastatic choriocarcinoma showing highly atypical cyto- and syncytiotrophoblastic cells.

Miscellanea—Other Metastatic Tumors *(continued)*

DIFFERENTIAL DIAGNOSIS

▪ The differential diagnosis of metastatic tumors to the breast may be problematic due to their frequent similarity to primary breast carcinoma.

▪ In metastatic cancer, DCIS is usually absent; in doubtful case, this criterion may raise further the index of suspicion about a metastasis, yet sporadic cases of metastases to the breast mimicking ductal carcinoma in situ have been reported.

▪ In males treated with hormone therapy for prostatic carcinoma (particularly ethynilestradiol- or diethylstilbestrol-based drugs), the breast may be colonized by small cell carcinoma or prostatic adenocarcinoma. Likely, hormone therapy in combination with a high-grade primary tumor represents a favoring factor.

▪ Metastatic tumors showing evidence of glandular differentiation, hence posing a serious differential diagnosis with infiltrating ductal carcinoma, may be the source of interpretive difficulties, especially on core needle biopsy specimens. A comprehensive clinical case evaluation followed by comparison of histologic findings are crucial to resolve the matter.

▪ Immunohistochemistry may be useful when a limited differential diagnosis is considered. ER and PR are usually strongly positive in well-to-moderately differentiated breast carcinomas, whereas other tumors such as kidney and lung carcinoma are not. Ovarian carcinoma may metastasize to the breast: this tumor is often positive for ER, yet a patchy rather than diffuse positivity is observed. Ovarian carcinoma is often positive for WT1. In addition, gastric and colorectal cancer may also exhibit ER and PR positivity. Lung adenocarcinoma is often positive for TTF1.

Miscellanea—Other Metastatic Tumors

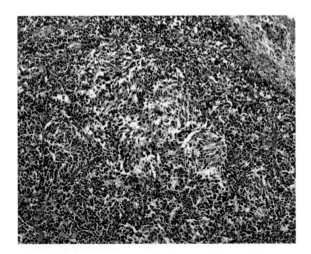

FIGURE 5-7
Metastatic medulloblastoma. Tumor
cells exhibit ribbons, festooning, and
rosette formation.

Lymphoma and Hematopoietic Disorders

DEFINITION
■ Lymphomas of breast are rare tumors primarily occurring in the mammary gland with or without involvement of ipsilateral axillary.
■ Some authors adopt less stringent criteria and allow including among breast lymphoma, tumors with a preponderant or initial involvement of the mammary gland which usually prove to be systemic diseases on further investigations.

CLINICAL FEATURES
■ Most cases of breast lymphomas are seen in postmenopausal patients and manifest as palpable masses. Multinodular lesions are not uncommon, and bilaterality has been reported in about 20% of cases. Bilaterality has also been described in puerperal women during lactation affected by Burkitt lymphoma. Another important condition is lymphoma that recurs, in the breast, as a secondary disease.
■ Mammography usually shows a roundish parenchymal opacity. Microcalcifications are absent. Abnormal mammograms are especially seen in low-grade lymphomas.
■ The prognosis of breast lymphoma does not differ from that of nodal lymphomas of comparable microscopic type and stage. There seems to be a relatively high frequency of cutaneous, soft tissue, bone, and brain recurrence.

GROSS FEATURES
■ Tumors appears as fleshy, poorly circumscribed masses. Regressive changes such as necrosis and hemorrhage may be recognized (Figure 5-8).

MICROSCOPIC FEATURES
■ Diffuse large B-cell lymphoma is the prevalent histologic type (Figure 5-9). Other forms include follicular lymphoma, Burkitt lymphoma, lymphoblastic lymphoma, anaplastic CD30+ lymphoma, and lymphomas of "mucosa-associated lymphoid tissue" type. A detailed microscopic description of breast lymphomas goes beyond the scope of this manual.
■ Large B-cell lymphoma presents as sheets of noncohesive, round to polygonal cells with variable amount of pale, sometimes plasmacytoid cytoplasm (Figure 5-10). Nuclei are vesicular and prominent nucleoli are common. Starry sky pattern of growths due to numerous macrophages may occasionally be observed. Indented or "cleaved" nuclei may be present as well. A brisk mitotic activity is common.
■ These tumors are characteristically positive for LCA, CD20 (Figure 5-11), CD79a, and negative for keratins. Frequently, there is a variable proportion of accompanying small T cells.

(continued)

Lymphoma and Hematopoietic Disorders

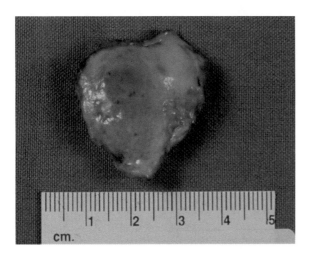

FIGURE 5-8
Gross specimen. Breast lymphoma presenting as a distinct nodule. Cut surface shows a tan, fish flesh-like, and glistening mass.

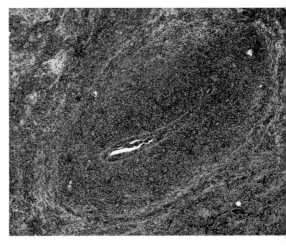

FIGURE 5-9
Large B-cell lymphoma of breast centered around a breast duct.

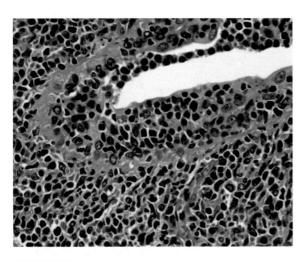

FIGURE 5-10
High-power view of large B-cell lymphoma. Tumor cells are comparable to those of follicular center cells and diffusely infiltrate the duct epithelium.

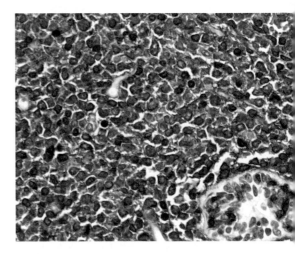

FIGURE 5-11
Strong immunoreactivity for CD20 of tumor cells of breast lymphoma.

Lymphoma and Hematopoietic Disorders *(continued)*

DIFFERENTIAL DIAGNOSIS

■ Breast lymphomas have to be differentiated mainly from poorly differentiated carcinoma due to their obviously different clinical implication. High-grade lobular carcinoma may be confused with lymphoma because of the discohesive proliferation of large cells, often with abundant stainable cytoplasm. Rare cases of anaplastic, large cell lymphoma may simulate medullary carcinoma. Application of immunohistochemistry is essential, yet, sometimes, it may be the source of interpretative errors if the entire clinicopathologic setting is not appreciated or only a few markers are applied. Some lymphomas may be positive for keratins or EMA (such as the anaplastic CD30+ lymphoma), and lymphoid markers may be exceptionally aberrantly expressed by some carcinomas.

■ Pseudolymphoma is a rare condition that may be difficult to distinguish from lymphoma grossly. Histologically, recognition of reactive follicular centers along with vascular proliferation aids in the distinction. Lymphocytoma cutis of the nipple due to *Borrelia burgdorferi* is a cause of breast lymphoid hyperplasia. Large, confluent germinal centers are often detected.

■ Extramedullary plasmacytoma may occur as a solitary breast nodule, hence mimicking breast cancer. The salient microscopic finding is a diffuse sheath of noncohesive round to oval nuclei with one or two peripheral nucleoli and abundant, stainable cytoplasm. Better differentiated tumors feature a cart-wheel chromatin pattern and a perinuclear halo. Poorly differentiated plasmacytic tumors show a more pronounced nuclear pleomorphism. Demonstration of CD138 positive cells with light chain restriction by means of antibodies directed against kappa or lambda light chains is useful for the diagnosis.

■ Rarely but not exceptionally, granulocytic sarcoma (chloroma) may present with breast involvement suggesting, among other possibilities, infiltration by a malignant lymphoma (Figure 5-12). In these cases, the distinction from lymphoma should be based on a careful evaluation of subtle microscopic details such as the indented or horseshoe shape of nuclei seen in metamyelocytic elements or the coarse cytoplasmic granularity of promyelocytes and myelocytes (Figure 5-13). Immunostaining for myeloperoxidase, CD34, and CD38 is a useful diagnostic aid.

■ Extramedullary myelopoiesis is another rare condition that may rarely present as a breast nodule, thus mimicking mammary carcinoma. Correct microscopic interpretation may be further compounded by the microscopic pattern featuring cells in disorderly array, including linear or small clusters resembling lobular carcinoma (Figure 5-14). However, rather than the monotonous cellularity seen in lobular carcinoma, or lymphoma, cell polymorphism is characteristically present due to the haphazard admixture of immature hemopoietic cells, including megakaryocytes and clusters of erythroid and nonnucleated red blood cells (Figure 5-15). Clinical correlation is critical, since these patients have evidence of systemic disorders including hepatomegaly and splenomegaly or abnormal peripheral blood counts on further medical evaluation. Abnormal bone marrow features are also often recognized.

■ Due to the relative rarity of these conditions, frozen section diagnosis is a potential source of serious mistakes and detrimental consequences to the patient.

Lymphoma and Hematopoietic Disorders

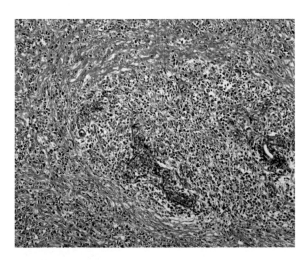

FIGURE 5-12
Granulocytic sarcoma of breast. This case was initially misinterpreted as large cell lymphoma.

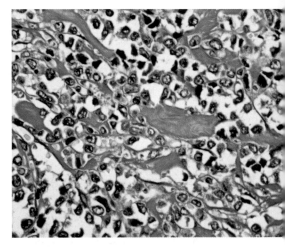

FIGURE 5-13
High-power view of granulocytic sarcoma showing a polymorphous infiltrate of tumor cells, some of which have a few cytoplasmic granules.

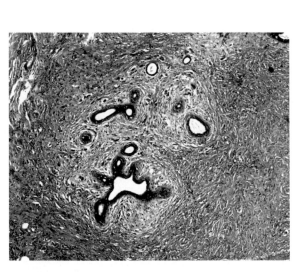

FIGURE 5-14
Extramedullary myelopoiesis of breast. The single cell infiltrate around preexisting breast units may deceitfully simulate infiltrating lobular carcinoma.

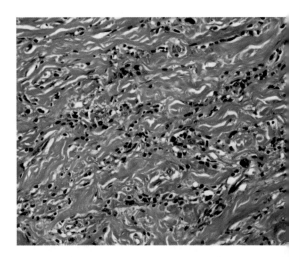

FIGURE 5-15
Details of extramedullary hematopoiesis. The infiltrate is polymorphous. Granulated hematopoietic elements are scattered in a linear pattern. Larger cells representing megakaryocytes may be recognized as well.

Appendix

OVERVIEW OF SENTINEL AND AXILLARY LYMPH NODE EVALUATION

DEFINITION

CLINICAL FEATURES

GROSS FEATURES

MICROSCOPIC FEATURES

DIFFERENTIAL DIAGNOSIS

REFERENCES

Overview of Sentinel and Axillary Lymph Node Evaluation

DEFINITION

Lymph nodes that can be involved by breast cancer metastasis include axillary, intramammary, internal mammary, supraclavicular, and infraclavicular lymph nodes. Axillary lymph nodes (ALN) include sentinel and nonsentinel lymph nodes. Most breast carcinomas drain to one or two sentinel nodes (SLN) that can be identified by the uptake of radiotracer, dye, or both. SLN is usually the first lymph node involved by metastasis and their involvement is highly predictive of non-SLN involvement. SLN biopsy can spare patients the increased morbidity of a complete ALN dissection.

CLINICAL FEATURES

The presence or absence of ALN metastases is the single most important traditional predictor of disease-free and overall survival, in breast cancer patients, in the absence of distant metastasis. Patients with positive lymph nodes have decreased disease-free and overall survival. With no lymph node involvement, the 10-year disease-free survival rate is close to 80%; the rate falls to 40% with one to three positive nodes and 15% in the presence of more than 10 positive nodes.

Currently, nearly 80% of mammographically detected breast cancers have negative ALN. For this reason, a less invasive sampling procedure, that is SLN biopsy, has rapidly replaced the traditional ALN dissection for evaluation of lymph nodes, accompanying excisional biopsy or mastectomy, in clinically node-negative invasive tumors. There are two main reasons why SLN biopsy has been adopted in routine clinical practice. Firstly, SLN metastases are more common than non-SLN metastases and secondly, ALN dissection is associated with significant morbidity including lymphedema, decreased range of motion, pain, and sensory loss. Because patients with a positive SLN have a high probability of having other positive non-SLN, a positive SLN biopsy is generally an indication for completion ALN dissection. A natural consequence of limited ALN sampling is that some patients require a two-stage ALN evaluation. SLN evaluation offers the potential to spare a large proportion of women the morbidity of an unnecessary ALN dissection.

Macrometastases (>2 mm) are of proven prognostic importance. The clinical significance of isolated tumor cells (ITC) and micrometastases, however, is unclear and is being addressed by current clinical trials. A number of single institution and observational studies and recent studies from two large randomized clinical trials (NSABP, B-32, and ACOSOG Z0011) have reported that patients with a negative SLN biopsy and no completion ALN dissection have very low locoregional failure rates. Furthermore, these studies also report that, the presence of small metastasis in SLN of clinically node-negative patients may not have a significant survival disadvantage.

GROSS FEATURES

There are no set numbers of lymph nodes that need to be found in a completion ALN dissection. However, many recommended at least 12 lymph nodes in each ALN dissection. The number of lymph nodes and their size range need to be recorded.

When a lymph node is positive on gross examination, a single representative tissue section is all that is required to confirm the diagnosis. This tissue section should include areas suspicious for extracapsular extension. Most lymph nodes, however, are negative on gross examination. These lymph nodes need to be submitted entirely for microscopic examination. In order to capture all macrometastatic deposits (>2 mm), it is recommended that lymph nodes be thinly sliced at 2-mm intervals and all slices submitted for microscopic evaluation. Care should be taken not to overcount the number of positive lymph nodes, by not submitting more than one serially sliced lymph nodes in one tissue cassette. If this has to be performed, each lymph node should be inked a different color for identification.

MICROSCOPIC FEATURES

A single H&E-stained surface section of each paraffin embedded block is all that is needed to capture all macrometastatic deposits, as long as the lymph nodes are sliced at not more than 2-mm intervals, and all slices submitted for microscopic evaluation. Immunohistochemical (IHC) staining may identify ITC within lymph nodes. However, the prognostic importance of these small metastases remains uncertain. The use of IHC may be useful in lobular carcinomas, where it may metastasize as single tumor cells and not as cohesive groups. In these cases, IHC may be used to better estimate the volume of metastatic deposits for nodal classification.

Intraoperative SLN evaluation is routinely performed in many institutions. Both frozen section and imprint cytology have been utilized intraoperatively with varying sensitivity and specificity. When a positive SLN is identified intraoperatively, an immediate completion ALN dissection is performed, in all patients. This is thought to help patients avoid a second operative procedure and a second anesthesia. However, when a positive SLN is first detected on a permanent section, completion ALN dissection may or may not be performed. In fact, most patients choose not to have completion ALN dissection, when all information is presented to them. This is because the decision, in these patients, is a multifactorial and multidisciplinary decision that considers not only the sentinel node status, but also the SLN nodal tumor burden, the number of SLN removed, primary tumor characteristics, and other patient factors. A study we conducted at the University of Vermont showed that, while intraoperative positive SLN leads to ALN dissection in 100% of patients, only 25% of patients choose to undergo ALN dissection when positive SLN is identified on permanent sections. These patients had mostly ITC and micrometastasis, but there were also patients with macrometastatic deposits. In this study (unpublished observation), we are suggesting that routine intraoperative SLN is not beneficial (may be harmful) to patients by having unnecessary ALN dissection.

Lymph node reporting should include the number of lymph nodes examined and the number of lymph nodes positive for metastasis. Also included in the report are the size of metastatic deposits with their classification (see below) and extra nodal extension. Lymph node metastases are classified based on the size of tumor deposits. Deposits >2 mm are classified as "macrometastasis," deposits >0.2 mm but not more than 2 mm are classified as "micrometastasis" (*AJCC 7th edition* also includes to micrometastasis, deposits of >200 tumor cells in a single cross section), and metastatic deposits not more than 0.2 mm are classified as "isolated tumor cells" (this also includes deposits <200 tumor cells—*AJCC 7th edition*).

In most cases, if metastases are present, the SLN will be the one that is involved. In rare cases, however, only non-SLN contains metastasis. These cases can occur if the true SLN is completely replaced by tumor (and therefore is not detected by radioactive tracer or dye),

Overview of Sentinel and Axillary Lymph Node Evaluation

if there is unusual lymphatic drainage, or if there is failure of the technique to identify the SLN.

DIFFERENTIAL DIAGNOSIS

Nevus cell aggregates, benign glandular inclusions, iatrogenic epithelial displacement, and lymphoma are rarely encountered in ALN. Close morphologic evaluation and IHC are helpful in distinguishing these findings from true metastasis. Nevus aggregates are positive for S-100, but negative for cytokeratins. Glandular inclusions may contain ciliated columnar epithelium and have different morphology than the primary carcinoma. Displaced epithelia usually originate from intraductal papillomas and are positive for myoepithelial markers.

REFERENCES

American Joint Committee on Cancer (AJCC) Staging Manual. 7th ed. Chicago, IL: Springer; 2009.

Bleiweiss IJ, Nagi CS, Jaffer S. Axillary sentinel lymph nodes can be falsely positive due to iatrogenic displacement and transport of benign epithelial cells in patients with breast carcinoma. *J Clin Oncol.* 2006;24(13):2013–2018.

Cserni G, Gregori D, Merletti F, et al. Meta-analysis of non-sentinel node metastases associated with micrometastasis sentinel nodes in breast cancer. *Br J Surg.* 2004;91(10):1245–1252.

Fisher ER, Anderson S, Redmond C, Fisher B. Pathologic findings from the National Surgical Adjuvant Breast Project protocol B-06. 10-year pathologic and clinical prognostic discriminates. *Cancer.* 1993;71(8):2507–2514.

Gipponi M, Bassetti C, Canavese G, et al. Sentinel lymph node as a new marker for therapeutic planning in breast cancer patients. *J Surg Oncol.* 2004;85(3):102–111.

Giuliano AE, Hunt KK, Ballman KV. Axillary dissection vs no axillary dissection in women with invasive breast cancer and sentinel node metastasis: a randomized clinical trial. *JAMA.* 2011;305(6):569–575.

Goyal A, Douglas-Jones A, Newcombe RG, Mansel RE. ALMANAC Trialists Group. Predictors of non-sentinel lymph node metastasis in breast cancer patients. *Eur J Cancer.* 2004;40(11):1731–1737.

Hack TF, Cohen L, Katz J, Robson LS, Goss P. Physical and psychological morbidity after axillary lymph node dissection for breast cancer. *J Clin Oncol.* 1999;17(1):143–149.

Hwang RF, Gonzalez-Angulo AM, Yi M, Buchholz TA, et al. Low locoregional failure rates in selected breast cancer patients with tumor-positive sentinel lymph nodes who do not undergo completion axillary dissection. *Cancer.* 2007;110(4):723–730.

Ivens D, Hoe AL, Podd TJ, Hamilton CR, Taylor I, Royle GT. Assessment of morbidity from complete axillary dissection. *Br J Cancer.* 1992;66(1):136–138.

Lyman GH, Giuliano AE, Somerfield MR, et al. American Society of Clinical Oncology guideline recommendations for sentinel lymph node biopsy in early-stage breast cancer. *J Clin Oncol.* 2005;23(30):7703–7720.

Maunsell E, Brisson J, Deschenes L. Arm problems and psychological distress after surgery for breast cancer. *Can J Surg.* 1993;36(4):315–320.

Naik AM, Fey J, Gemignani M, et al. The risk of axillary relapse after sentinel lymph node biopsy for breast cancer is comparable with that of axillary lymph node dissection: a follow-up study of 4008 procedures. *Ann Surg.* 2004;240(3):462–468; discussion 468–471.

Norton LE, Komenaka IK, Emerson RE, Murphy C, Badve S. Benign glandular inclusions a rare cause of a false positive sentinel node. *J Surg Oncol.* 2007;95(7):593–596.

Overview of Sentinel and Axillary Lymph Node Evaluation

Peng Y, Ashfaq R, Ewing G, Leitch AM, Molberg KH. False-positive sentinel lymph nodes in breast cancer patients caused by benign glandular inclusions: report of three cases and review of the literature. *Am J Clin Pathol.* 2008;130(1):21–27; quiz 146.

Pizzolitto S, Gentile G. Comprehensive examination of sentinel lymph node in breast cancer: a solution without a problem? Int J Surg Pathol 2006;14:1-8.

Roses DF, Brooks AD, Harris MN, Shapiro RL, Mitnick J. Complications of level I and II axillary dissection in the treatment of carcinoma of the breast. *Ann Surg.* 1999;230(2):194–201.

Russo J, Frederick J, Ownby HE, et al. Predictors of recurrence and survival of patients with breast cancer. *Am J Clin Pathol.* 1987;88(2):123–131.

Schwartz GF. Clinical practice guidelines for the use of axillary sentinel lymph node biopsy in carcinoma of the breast: current update. *Breast J.* 2004;10(2):85–88.

Schwartz GF, Giuliano AE, Veronesi U. Consensus Conference Committee. Proceedings of the consensus conference on the role of sentinel lymph node biopsy in carcinoma of the breast April 19 to 22, 2001, Philadelphia, Pennsylvania. *Hum Pathol.* 2002;33(6):579–589.

Velanovich V, Szymanski W. Quality of life of breast cancer patients with lymphedema. *Am J Surg.* 1999;177(3):184–187; discussion 188.

Weaver DL, Rosenberg RD, Barlow WE, et al. Pathologic findings from the Breast Cancer Surveillance Consortium: population-based outcomes in women undergoing biopsy after screening mammography. *Cancer.* 2006;106(4):732–242.

Weaver DL, Ashikaga T, Krag DN, et al. Effect of occult metastases on survival in node-negative breast cancer. *N Engl J Med* 2011;364:412–421.

Weaver DL. Pathology evaluation of sentinel lymph nodes in breast cancer: protocol recommendations and rationale. *Mod Pathol.* 2010;23(suppl 2):S26–S32.

Wong SL, Edwards MJ, Chao C, et al. The effect of lymphatic tumor burden on sentinel lymph node biopsy results. *Breast J.* 2002;8(4):192–198.

References

1. COMMON BENIGN CONDITIONS

FIBROCYSTIC CHANGES

Durham JR, Fechner RE. The histologic spectrum of apocrine lesions of the breast. *Am J Clin Pathol.* 2000;113:S3–S18.

Eusebi V, Foschini MP, Betts CM, et al. Microglandular adenosis, apocrine adenosis, and tubular carcinoma of the breast. An immunohistochemical comparison. *Am J Surg Pathol.* 1993;17:99–109.

Masood S, Rosa M. The challenge of apocrine proliferations of the breast: a morphologic approach. *Pathol Res Pract.* 2009;205:155–164.

Wells CA, El-Ayat GA. Non-operative breast pathology: apocrine lesions. *J Clin Pathol.* 2007;60:1313–1320.

PERIDUCTAL MASTITIS
(DUCT ECTASIA)

Ammari FF, Yaghan RJ, Omari AK. Periductal mastitis. Clinical characteristics and outcome. *Saudi Med J.* 2002;23:819–822.

Dixon JM. Periductal mastitis/duct ectasia. *World J Surg.* 1989;13:715–720.

Dixon JM, Ravisekar O, Chetty U, et al. Periductal mastitis and duct ectasia: different conditions with different aetiologies. *Br J Surg.* 1996;83:820–822.

Furlong AJ, al-Nakib L, Knox WF, et al. Periductal inflammation and cigarette smoke. *J Am Coll Surg.* 1994;179:417–420.

Miller SD, McCollough ML, DeNapoli T. Periductal mastitis. Masquerading as carcinoma. *Dermatol Surg.* 1998;24:383–385.

Nicholson BT, Harvey JA, Cohen MA. Nipple-areolar complex: normal anatomy and benign and malignant processes. *Radiographics.* 2009;29:509–523.

FAT NECROSIS

Azzopardi JG, Ahmed A, Millis RR. *Problems in Breast Pathology.* Philadelphia, PA: Saunders; 1979.

Bilgen IG, Ustun EE, Memis A. Fat necrosis of the breast: clinical, mammographic and sonographic features. *Eur J Radiol.* 2001;39:92–99.

Daly CP, Jaeger B, Sill DS. Variable appearances of fat necrosis on breast MRI. *AJR Am J Roentgenol.* 2008;191:1374–1380.

Ganau S, Tortajada L, Escribano F, et al. The great mimicker: fat necrosis of the breast–magnetic resonance mammography approach. *Curr Probl Diagn Radiol.* 2009;38:189–197.

Haj M, Loberant N, Salamon V, et al. Membranous fat necrosis of the breast: diagnosis by minimally invasive technique. *Breast J.* 2004;10:504–508.

Poppiti RJ Jr, Margulies M, Cabello B, et al. Membranous fat necrosis. *Am J Surg Pathol.* 1986;10:62–69.

Pullyblank AM, Davies JD, Basten J, et al. Fat necrosis of the female breast–Hadfield re-visited. *Breast.* 2001;10:388–391.

Taboada JL, Stephens TW, Krishnamurthy S, et al. The many faces of fat necrosis in the breast. *AJR Am J Roentgenol.* 2009;192:815–825.

SILICON MASTITIS

Axelsen RA, Reasbeck P. Granulomatous lobular mastitis: report of a case with previously undescribed histopathological abnormalities. *Pathology.* 1988;20:383–389.

Backovic A, Wolfram D. Silicone mammary implants–can we turn back the time? *Exp Gerontol.* 2007;42:713–718.

Bassler R, Birke F. Histopathology of tumour associated sarcoid-like stromal reaction in breast cancer. An analysis of 5 cases with immunohistochemical investigations. *Virchows Arch A Pathol Anat Histopathol.* 1988;412:231–239.

Brickman M, Parsa NN, Parsa FD. Late hematoma after breast implantation. *Aesthetic Plast Surg.* 2004;28:80–82.

Fong D, Lann MA, Finlayson C, et al. Diabetic (lymphocytic) mastopathy with exuberant lympho-histiocytic and granulomatous response: a case report with review of the literature. *Am J Surg Pathol.* 2006;30:1330–1336.

Galea MH, Robertson JF, Ellis IO, et al. Granulomatous lobular mastitis. *Aust N Z J Surg.* 1989;59:547–550.

Giron GL, Tartter PI. Image of the month. Silicone mastitis with abscess. *Arch Surg.* 2004;139:341–342.

Kessler W, Wolloch Y. Granulomatous mastitis. A lesion clinically simulating carcinoma. *Am J Clin Pathol.* 1972;58:642–646.

Ko C, Ahn CY, Markowitz BL. Injected liquid silicone, chronic mastitis, and undetected breast cancer. *Ann Plast Surg.* 1995;34:176–179.

Newman MK, Zemmel NJ, Bandak AZ, et al. Primary breast lymphoma in a patient with silicone breast implants: a case report and review of the literature. *J Plast Reconstr Aesthet Surg.* 2008;61:822–825.

Poeppl N, Schreml S, Lichtenegger F, et al. Does the surface structure of implants have an impact on the formation of a capsular contracture? *Aesthetic Plast Surg.* 2007;31:133–139.

Yoshida SH, Swan S, Teuber SS, et al. Silicone breast implants: immunotoxic and epidemiologic issues. *Life Sci.* 1995;56:1299–1310.

PREGNANCY/HORMONE RELATED CHANGES

Battersby S, Anderson TJ. Histological changes in breast tissue that characterize recent pregnancy. *Histopathology.* 1989;15:415–419.

Kiaer HW, Andersen JA. Focal pregnancy-like changes in the breast. *Acta Pathol Microbiol Scand A.* 1977;85:931–941.

Page DL, Anderson TJ. *Diagnostic Histopathology of the Breast.* Edinburgh, NY: Churchill Livingstone; 1987.

Rosen PP. *Rosen's breast pathology,* 3rd ed. Philadelphia, PA: Lippincott Williams & Wilkins; 2008.

Tavassoli FA, Yeh IT. Lactational and clear cell changes of the breast in nonlactating, nonpregnant women. *Am J Clin Pathol.* 1987;87:23–29.

DIABETIC MASTOPATHY

Allen PW, Fisher C. Selected case from the Arkadi M. Rywlin International Pathology Slide Seminar: diabetic mastopathy. *Adv Anat Pathol.* 2001;8:298–301.

Dixon JM, Ravisekar O, Chetty U, et al. Periductal mastitis and duct ectasia: different conditions with different aetiologies. *Br J Surg.* 1996;83:820–822.

Ely KA, Tse G, Simpson JF, et al. Diabetic mastopathy. A clinicopathologic review. *Am J Clin Pathol.* 2000;113:541–545.

Fong D, Lann MA, Finlayson C, et al. Diabetic (lymphocytic) mastopathy with exuberant lympho-histiocytic and granulomatous response: a case report with review of the literature. *Am J Surg Pathol.* 2006;30.1330–1336.

Foschini MP, Cavazza A, Macedo Pinto IM, et al. Diabetic fibrous mastopathy. Report of two cases. *Virchows Arch A Pathol Anat Histopathol.* 1990;417:529–532.

Haj M, Loberant N, Salamon V, et al. Membranous fat necrosis of the breast: diagnosis by minimally invasive technique. *Breast J.* 2004;10:504–508.

Hunfeld KP, Bassler R, Kronsbein H. "Diabetic mastopathy" in the male breast–a special type of gynecomastia. A comparative study of lymphocytic mastitis and gynecomastia. *Pathol Res Pract.* 1997;193:197–205.

Kudva YC, Reynolds C, O'Brien T, et al. "Diabetic mastopathy," or sclerosing lymphocytic lobulitis, is strongly associated with type 1 diabetes. *Diabetes Care.* 2002;25:121–126.

Kudva YC, Reynolds CA, O'Brien T, et al. Mastopathy and diabetes. *Curr Diab Rep.* 2003;3:56–59.

Pereira MA, de Magalhaes AV, da Motta LD, et al. Fibrous mastopathy: clinical, imaging, and histopathologic findings of 31 cases. *J Obstet Gynaecol Res.* 2010;36:326–335.

Poppiti RJ Jr, Margulies M, Cabello B, et al. Membranous fat necrosis. *Am J Surg Pathol.* 1986;10:62–69.

Shousha S. Diabetic mastopathy: strong CD10+ immunoreactivity of the atypical stromal cells. *Histopathology.* 2008;52:648–650.

Talele AC, Slanetz PJ, Edmister WB, et al. The lactating breast: MRI findings and literature review. *Breast J.* 2003;9:237–240.

Thorncroft K, Forsyth L, Desmond S, et al. The diagnosis and management of diabetic mastopathy. *Breast J.* 2007;13:607–613.

Tomaszewski JE, Brooks JS, Hicks D, et al. Diabetic mastopathy: a distinctive clinicopathologic entity. *Hum Pathol.* 1992;23:780–786.

Valdez R, Thorson J, Finn WG, et al. Lymphocytic mastitis and diabetic mastopathy: a molecular, immunophenotypic, and clinicopathologic evaluation of 11 cases. *Mod Pathol.* 2003;16:223–228.

Yamashita M, Ogawa T, Hanamura N, et al. An uncommon case of T1b breast cancer with diabetic mastopathy in type II diabetes mellitus. *Breast Cancer.* 2009; Sep 30 2009 epub.

ADENOSIS

Azzopardi JG, Ahmed A, Millis RR: Problems in breast pathology. Phildelphia, PA: Saunders, 1979. (*Major Problems in Pathology* v. 11).

Dupont WD, Page DL. Risk factors for breast cancer in women with proliferative breast disease. *N Engl J Med.* 1985;312:146–151.

Kalof AN, Tam D, Beatty B, Cooper K. Immunostaining patterns of myoepithelial cells in breast lesions: a comparison of CD10 and smooth muscle myosin heavy chain. *J Clin Pathol.* 2004;57: 625–629.

Lee KC, Chan JK, Gwi E. Tubular adenosis of the breast. A distinctive benign lesion mimicking invasive carcinoma. *Am J Surg Pathol.* 1996;20:46–54.

Nielsen BB. Adenosis tumour of the breast—a clinicopathological investigation of 27 cases. *Histopathology.* 1987;11:1259–1275.

Page DL, Anderson TJ. *Diagnostic histopathology of the breast.* Edinburgh; NY: Churchill Livingstone, 1987.

Rosen PP, Hoda SA. *Breast pathology: Diagnosis by needle core biopsy, 3rd ed.* Philadelphia, PA: Wolters Kluwer/Lippincott Williams & Wilkins Health, 2010.

SPECIAL TYPES OF ADENOSIS: Sclerosing Adenosis

Azzopardi JG, Ahmed A, Millis RR. *Problems in breast pathology.* Phildelphia, PA: Saunders, 1979. (*Major Problems in Pathology* v. 11).

Chen YB, Magpayo J, Rosen PP. Sclerosing adenosis in sentinel axillary lymph nodes from a patient with invasive ductal carcinoma: an unusual variant of benign glandular inclusions. *Arch Pathol Lab Med.* 2008;132:1439–1441.

Fechner RE. Lobular carcinoma in situ in sclerosing adenosis. A potential source of confusion with invasive carcinoma. *Am J Surg Pathol.*1981;5:233–239.

Jensen RA, Page DL, Dupont WD, Rogers LW. Invasive breast cancer risk in women with sclerosing adenosis. *Cancer*. 1989;64:1977–1983.

MacErlean DP, Nathan BE. Calcification in sclerosing adenosis simulating malignant breast calcification. *Br J Radiol*. 1972;45:944–945.

Page DL, Anderson TJ. *Diagnostic histopathology of the breast*. Edinburgh, NY: Churchill Livingstone, 1987.

SPECIAL TYPES OF ADENOSIS: Microglandular Adenosis

Eusebi V, Foschini MP, Betts CM, Gherardi G, Millis RR, Bussolati G, Azzopardi JG. Microglandular adenosis, apocrine adenosis, and tubular carcinoma of the breast. An immunohistochemical comparison. *Am J Surg Pathol*. 1993;17:99–109.

Khalifeh IM, Albarracin C, Diaz LK, Symmans FW, Edgerton ME, Hwang RF, Sneige N. Clinical, histopathologic, and immunohistochemical features of microglandular adenosis and transition into in situ and invasive carcinoma. *Am J Surg Pathol*. 2008;32:544–552.

Rosen PP. Microglandular adenosis. A benign lesion simulating invasive mammary carcinoma. *Am J Surg Pathol*. 1983;7:137–144.

Rosen PP, Hoda SA. *Breast pathology: Diagnosis by needle core biopsy*, 3rd ed. Philadelphia, PA: Wolters Kluwer/Lippincott Williams & Wilkins Health, 2010, pp 61–76.

Rosenblum MK, Purrazzella R, Rosen PP. Is microglandular adenosis a precancerous disease? A study of carcinoma arising therein. *Am J Surg Pathol*. 1986;10:237–245.

Salarieh A, Sneige N. Breast carcinoma arising in microglandular adenosis: a review of the literature. *Arch Pathol Lab Med*. 2007;131:1397–1399.

2. PROLIFERATIVE AND PREINVASIVE EPITHELIAL LESIONS

USUAL DUCTAL HYPERPLASIA

Azzopardi JG, Ahmed A, Millis RR. *Problems in Breast Pathology*. Philadelphia, PA: Saunders; 1979.

Bianchi S, Palli D, Galli M, et al. Benign breast disease and cancer risk. *Crit Rev Oncol Hematol*. 1993;15:221–242.

Dupont WD, Page DL. Risk factors for breast cancer in women with proliferative breast disease. *N Engl J Med*. 1985;312:146–151.

Schnitt SJ. Benign breast disease and breast cancer risk: morphology and beyond. *Am J Surg Pathol*. 2003;27:836–841.

ATYPICAL DUCTAL HYPERPLASIA

Bianchi S, Palli D, Galli M, et al. Benign breast disease and cancer risk. *Crit Rev Oncol Hematol*. 1993;15:221–242.

Dupont WD, Parl FF, Hartmann WH, et al. Breast cancer risk associated with proliferative breast disease and atypical hyperplasia. *Cancer*. 1993;71:1258–1265.

Marshall LM, Hunter DJ, Connolly JL, et al. Risk of breast cancer associated with atypical hyperplasia of lobular and ductal types. *Cancer Epidemiol Biomarkers Prev*. 1997;6:297–301.

Page DL, Dupont WD, Rogers LW, et al. Atypical hyperplastic lesions of the female breast. A long-term follow-up study. *Cancer*. 1985;55:2698–2708.

Pinder SE, Ellis IO. The diagnosis and management of pre-invasive breast disease: ductal carcinoma in situ (DCIS) and atypical ductal hyperplasia (ADH)–current definitions and classification. *Breast Cancer Res*. 2003;5:254–257.

Rosai J. Borderline epithelial lesions of the breast. *Am J Surg Pathol*. 1991;15:209–221.

Schnitt SJ, Connolly JL, Tavassoli FA, et al. Interobserver reproducibility in the diagnosis of ductal proliferative breast lesions using standardized criteria. *Am J Surg Pathol*. 1992;16:1133–1143.

Simpson JF. Update on atypical epithelial hyperplasia and ductal carcinoma in situ. *Pathology*. 2009;41:36–39.

Zagouri F, Sergentanis TN, Zografos GC. Precursors and preinvasive lesions of the breast: the role of molecular prognostic markers in the diagnostic and therapeutic dilemma. *World J Surg Oncol.* 2007;5:57.

COLUMNAR CELL LESIONS

Aulmann S, Elsawaf Z, Penzel R, et al. Invasive tubular carcinoma of the breast frequently is clonally related to flat epithelial atypia and low-grade ductal carcinoma in situ. *Am J Surg Pathol.* 2009;33:1646–1653.

Azzopardi JG, Ahmed A, Millis RR. *Problems in Breast Pathology.* Philadelphia, PA: Saunders; 1979.

Feeley L, Quinn CM. Columnar cell lesions of the breast. *Histopathology.* 2008;52:11–19.

Lerwill MF. Flat epithelial atypia of the breast. *Arch Pathol Lab Med.* 2008;132:615–621.

Moinfar F. Flat ductal intraepithelial neoplasia of the breast: a review of diagnostic criteria, differential diagnoses, molecular-genetic findings, and clinical relevance—it is time to appreciate the Azzopardi concept! *Arch Pathol Lab Med.* 2009;133:879–892.

Schnitt SJ, Vincent-Salomon A. Columnar cell lesions of the breast. *Adv Anat Pathol.* 2003;10:113–124.

Simpson PT, Gale T, Reis-Filho JS, et al. Columnar cell lesions of the breast: the missing link in breast cancer progression? A morphological and molecular analysis. *Am J Surg Pathol.* 2005;29:734–746.

Tavassoli FA, Devilee P, International Agency for Research on Cancer, et al. *Pathology and Genetics of Tumours of the Breast and Female Genital Organs.* Lyon, France: IARC Press; 2003.

DUCTAL CARCINOMA IN SITU

NHS BSP Publications. Classifying epithelial proliferation. In: *Pathology Reporting in Breast Cancer Screening: National Coordinating Group for Breast Screening.* 2nd ed. NHS BSP Publications; 1995.

Azzopardi JG, Ahmed A, Millis RR. *Problems in Breast Pathology.* Philadelphia, PA: Saunders; 1979.

Dupont WD, Page DL. Risk factors for breast cancer in women with proliferative breast disease. *N Engl J Med.* 1985;312:146–151.

Ellis IO, Pinder SE, Lee AH, et al. A critical appraisal of existing classification systems of epithelial hyperplasia and in situ neoplasia of the breast with proposals for future methods of categorization: where are we going? *Semin Diagn Pathol.* 1999;16:202–208.

Page DL, Anderson TJ. *Diagnostic Histopathology of the Breast.* Edinburgh, NY: Churchill Livingstone; 1987.

Rosai J. Borderline epithelial lesions of the breast. *Am J Surg Pathol.* 1991;15:209–221.

Schnitt SJ, Connolly JL, Tavassoli FA, et al. Interobserver reproducibility in the diagnosis of ductal proliferative breast lesions using standardized criteria. *Am J Surg Pathol.* 1992;16:1133–1143.

Simpson JF. Update on atypical epithelial hyperplasia and ductal carcinoma in situ. *Pathology.* 2009;41:36–39.

Tavassoli FA, Devilee P, International Agency for Research on Cancer, et al. *Pathology and Genetics of Tumours of the Breast and Female Genital Organs.* Lyon, France: IARC Press; 2003.

LOBULAR NEOPLASIA

Barsky SH, Bose S. Should LCIS be regarded as a heterogeneous disease? *Breast J.* 1999;5:407–412.

Bentz JS, Yassa N, Clayton F. Pleomorphic lobular carcinoma of the breast: clinicopathologic features of 12 cases. *Mod Pathol.* 1998;11:814–822.

Cangiarella J, Guth A, Axelrod D, et al. Is surgical excision necessary for the management of atypical lobular hyperplasia and lobular carcinoma in situ diagnosed on core needle biopsy?: a report of 38 cases and review of the literature. *Arch Pathol Lab Med.* 2008;132:979–983.

Chen YY, Hwang ES, Roy R, et al. Genetic and phenotypic characteristics of pleomorphic lobular carcinoma in situ of the breast. *Am J Surg Pathol.* 2009;33:1683–1694.

Chivukula M, Haynik DM, Brufsky A, et al. Pleomorphic lobular carcinoma in situ (PLCIS) on breast core needle biopsies: clinical significance and immunoprofile. *Am J Surg Pathol.* 2008;32:1721–1726.

Contreras A, Sattar H. Lobular neoplasia of the breast: an update. *Arch Pathol Lab Med.* 2009;133:1116–1120.

Da Silva L, Parry S, Reid L, et al. Aberrant expression of E-cadherin in lobular carcinomas of the breast. *Am J Surg Pathol.* 2008;32:773–783.

Fadare O, Dadmanesh F, Alvarado-Cabrero I, et al. Lobular intraepithelial neoplasia [lobular carcinoma in situ] with comedo-type necrosis: A clinicopathologic study of 18 cases. *Am J Surg Pathol.* 2006;30:1445–1453.

Foote FW, Stewart FW. Lobular carcinoma in situ: a rare form of mammary cancer. *Am J Pathol.* 1941;17:491–463.

Jacobs TW, Pliss N, Kouria G, et al. Carcinomas in situ of the breast with indeterminate features: role of E-cadherin staining in categorization. *Am J Surg Pathol.* 2001;25:229–236.

Menon S, Porter GJ, Evans AJ, et al. The significance of lobular neoplasia on needle core biopsy of the breast. *Virchows Arch.* 2008;452:473–479.

Middleton LP, Palacios DM, Bryant BR, et al. Pleomorphic lobular carcinoma: morphology, immuno-histochemistry, and molecular analysis. *Am J Surg Pathol.* 2000;24:1650–1656.

Schnitt SJ, Morrow M. Lobular carcinoma in situ: current concepts and controversies. *Semin Diagn Pathol.* 1999;16:209–223.

Sgroi D, Koerner FC. Involvement of collagenous spherulosis by lobular carcinoma in situ. Potential confusion with cribriform ductal carcinoma in situ. *Am J Surg Pathol.* 1995;19:1366–1370.

Wahed A, Connelly J, Reese T. E-cadherin expression in pleomorphic lobular carcinoma: an aid to differentiation from ductal carcinoma. *Ann Diagn Pathol.* 2002;6:349–351.

PAPILLOMA AND PAPILLOMATOSIS

Azzopardi JG, Ahmed A, Millis RR. *Problems in Breast Pathology.* Philadelphia, PA: Saunders; 1979.

Collins LC, Schnitt SJ. Papillary lesions of the breast: selected diagnostic and management issues. *Histopathology.* 2008;52:20–29.

de Moraes Schenka NG, Schenka AA, de Souza Queiroz L, et al. Use of p63 and CD10 in the differen-tial diagnosis of papillary neoplasms of the breast. *Breast J.* 2008;14:68–75.

Kihara M, Miyauchi A. Intracystic papilloma of the breast forming a giant cyst. *Breast Cancer.* 2010;17:68–70.

Koerner F. Papilloma and papillary carcinoma. *Semin Diagn Pathol.* 2010;27:13–30.

Mulligan AM, O'Malley FP. Papillary lesions of the breast: a review. *Adv Anat Pathol.* 2007;14:108–119.

Page DL, Salhany KE, Jensen RA, et al. Subsequent breast carcinoma risk after biopsy with atypia in a breast papilloma. *Cancer.* 1996;78:258–266.

Rosen PP, Cantrell B, Mullen DL, et al. Juvenile papillomatosis (Swiss cheese disease) of the breast. *Am J Surg Pathol.* 1980;4:3–12.

Rosen PP, Kimmel M. Juvenile papillomatosis of the breast. A follow-up study of 41 patients having biopsies before 1979. *Am J Clin Pathol.* 1990;93:599–603.

Tavassoli FA, Devilee P, International Agency for Research on Cancer, et al. *Pathology and Genetics of Tumours of the Breast and Female Genital Organs.* Lyon, France: IARC Press; 2003.

Tse GM, Tan PH, Lui PC, et al. The role of immunohistochemistry for smooth-muscle actin, p63, CD10 and cytokeratin 14 in the differential diagnosis of papillary lesions of the breast. *J Clin Pathol.* 2007;60:315–320.

Tse GM, Tan PH, Moriya T. The role of immunohistochemistry in the differential diagnosis of papillary lesions of the breast. *J Clin Pathol.* 2009;62:407–413.

Ueng SH, Mezzetti T, Tavassoli FA. Papillary neoplasms of the breast: a review. *Arch Pathol Lab Med.* 2009;133:893–907.

NIPPLE ADENOMA

Perzin KH, Lattes R. Papillary adenoma of the nipple (florid papillomatosis, adenoma, adenomatosis). A clinicopathologic study. *Cancer.* 1972;29:996–1009.

Rosen PP, Caicco JA. Florid papillomatosis of the nipple. A study of 51 patients, including nine with mammary carcinoma. *Am J Surg Pathol.* 1986;10:87–101.

Tavassoli FA, Devilee P, International Agency for Research on Cancer, et al. *Pathology and Genetics of Tumours of the Breast and Female Genital Organs.* Lyon, France: IARC Press; 2003.

COMPLEX SCLEROSING LESIONS/RADIAL SCAR

Brenner RJ, Jackman RJ, Parker SH, et al. Percutaneous core needle biopsy of radial scars of the breast: when is excision necessary? *AJR Am J Roentgenol.* 2002;179:1179–1184.

Eusebi V, Millis RR. Epitheliosis, infiltrating epitheliosis, and radial scar. *Semin Diagn Pathol.* 2010;27:5–12.

Jacobs TW, Byrne C, Colditz G, et al. Radial scars in benign breast-biopsy specimens and the risk of breast cancer. *N Engl J Med.* 1999;340:430–436.

Kalof AN, Tam D, Beatty B, et al. Immunostaining patterns of myoepithelial cells in breast lesions: a comparison of CD10 and smooth muscle myosin heavy chain. *J Clin Pathol.* 2004;57:625–629.

Kennedy M, Masterson AV, Kerin M, et al. Pathology and clinical relevance of radial scars: a review. *J Clin Pathol.* 2003;56:721–724.

Noel JC, Fayt I, Fernandez-Aguilar S. [P63 protein in the diagnosis of breast tubular carcinoma]. *Ann Pathol.* 2004;24:319–323.

3. INVASIVE CARCINOMAS

USUAL INVASIVE DUCTAL CARCINOMA (OR INFILTRATING CARCINOMA, NOS)

Barbareschi M, Pecciarini L, Cangi MG, et al. p63, a p53 homologue, is a selective nuclear marker of myoepithelial cells of the human breast. *Am J Surg Pathol.* 2001;25:1054–1060.

Ellis IO, Galea M, Broughton N, et al. Pathological prognostic factors in breast cancer. II. Histological type. Relationship with survival in a large study with long-term follow-up. *Histopathology.* 1992;20:479–489.

Elston CW, Ellis IO. Pathological prognostic factors in breast cancer. I. The value of histological grade in breast cancer: experience from a large study with long-term follow-up. *Histopathology.* 1991;19:403–410.

Fisher CJ, Egan MK, Smith P, et al. Histopathology of breast cancer in relation to age. *Br J Cancer.* 1997;75:593–596.

Fisher ER, Palekar AS, Redmond C, et al. Pathologic findings from the National Surgical Adjuvant Breast Project (protocol no. 4). VI. Invasive papillary cancer. *Am J Clin Pathol.* 1980;73:313–322.

Page DL, Anderson TJ. *Diagnostic Histopathology of the Breast.* Edinburgh, NY: Churchill Livingstone; 1987.

Robbins P, Pinder S, de Klerk N, et al. Histological grading of breast carcinomas: a study of interobserver agreement. *Hum Pathol.* 1995;26:873–879.

Tavassoli FA, Eusebi V, American Registry of Pathology, et al. *Tumors of the Mammary Gland.* Washington, D.C.: American Registry of Pathology in collaboration with the Armed Forces Institute of Pathology; 2009.

INFILTRATING LOBULAR CARCINOMA

Fisher ER, Fisher B. Lobular carcinoma of the breast: an overview. *Ann Surg.* 1977;185:377–385.

Giffler RF, Kay S. Small-cell carcinoma of the male mammary gland. A tumor resembling infiltrating lobular carcinoma. *Am J Clin Pathol.* 1976;66:715–722.

Harris M, Howell A, Chrissohou M, et al. A comparison of the metastatic pattern of infiltrating lobular carcinoma and infiltrating duct carcinoma of the breast. *Br J Cancer.* 1984;50:23–30.

Hilleren DJ, Andersson IT, Lindholm K, et al. Invasive lobular carcinoma: mammographic findings in a 10-year experience. *Radiology.* 1991;178:149–154.

Lamovec J, Bracko M. Metastatic pattern of infiltrating lobular carcinoma of the breast: an autopsy study. *J Surg Oncol.* 1991;48:28–33.

Papotti M, Gherardi G, Eusebi V, et al. Primary oat cell (neuroendocrine) carcinoma of the breast. Report of four cases. *Virchows Arch A Pathol Anat Histopathol.* 1992;420:103–108.

Rakha EA, Patel A, Powe DG, et al. Clinical and biological significance of E-cadherin protein expression in invasive lobular carcinoma of the breast. *Am J Surg Pathol.* 2010;34:1472–1479.

Reis-Filho JS, Simpson PT, Jones C, et al. Pleomorphic lobular carcinoma of the breast: role of comprehensive molecular pathology in characterization of an entity. *J Pathol.* 2005;207:1–13.

Rosen PP, Hoda SA, Dershaw DD, et al. *Breast Pathology: Diagnosis by Needle Core Biopsy.* 2nd ed. Philadelphia, PA: Lippincott Williams & Wilkins; 2006.

Shin SJ, DeLellis RA, Ying L, et al. Small cell carcinoma of the breast: a clinicopathologic and immunohistochemical study of nine patients. *Am J Surg Pathol.* 2000;24:1231–1238.

Wheeler JE, Enterline HT. Lobular carcinoma of the breast in situ and infiltrating. *Pathol Annu.* 1976;11:161–188.

TUBULAR CARCINOMA

Diab SG, Clark GM, Osborne CK, et al. Tumor characteristics and clinical outcome of tubular and mucinous breast carcinomas. *J Clin Oncol.* 1999;17:1442–1448.

Ellis IO, Galea M, Broughton N, et al. Pathological prognostic factors in breast cancer. II. Histological type. Relationship with survival in a large study with long-term follow-up. *Histopathology.* 1992;20:479–489.

Gottlieb C, Raju U, Greenwald KA. Myoepithelial cells in the differential diagnosis of complex benign and malignant breast lesions: an immunohistochemical study. *Mod Pathol.* 1990;3: 135–140.

Lerwill MF. Flat epithelial atypia of the breast. *Arch Pathol Lab Med.* 2008;132:615–621.

Mastropasqua MG, Maiorano E, Pruneri G, et al. Immunoreactivity for c-kit and p63 as an adjunct in the diagnosis of adenoid cystic carcinoma of the breast. *Mod Pathol.* 2005;18:1277–1282.

Mitnick JS, Gianutsos R, Pollack AH, et al. Tubular carcinoma of the breast: sensitivity of diagnostic techniques and correlation with histopathology. *AJR Am J Roentgenol.* 1999;172:319–323.

Rosen PP, Hoda SA, Dershaw DD, et al. *Breast Pathology: Diagnosis by Needle Core Biopsy.* 2nd ed. Philadelphia, PA: Lippincott Williams & Wilkins; 2006.

Tavassoli FA, Eusebi V, American Registry of Pathology, et al. *Tumors of the Mammary Gland.* Washington, D.C.: American Registry of Pathology in collaboration with the Armed Forces Institute of Pathology; 2009.

Tavassoli FA, Norris HJ. Microglandular adenosis of the breast. A clinicopathologic study of 11 cases with ultrastructural observations. *Am J Surg Pathol.* 1983;7:731–737.

Tobon H, Salazar H. Tubular carcinoma of the breast. Clinical, histological, and ultrastructural observations. *Arch Pathol Lab Med.* 1977;101:310–316.

MUCINOUS CARCINOMA

Capella C, Eusebi V, Mann B, et al. Endocrine differentiation in mucoid carcinoma of the breast. *Histopathology.* 1980;4:613–630.

Clayton F. Pure mucinous carcinomas of breast: morphologic features and prognostic correlates. *Hum Pathol.* 1986;17:34–38.

Diab SG, Clark GM, Osborne CK, et al. Tumor characteristics and clinical outcome of tubular and mucinous breast carcinomas. *J Clin Oncol.* 1999;17:1442–1448.

Ellis IO, Galea M, Broughton N, et al. Pathological prognostic factors in breast cancer. II. Histological type. Relationship with survival in a large study with long-term follow-up. *Histopathology.* 1992;20:479–489.

Komaki K, Sakamoto G, Sugano H, et al. Mucinous carcinoma of the breast in Japan. A prognostic analysis based on morphologic features. *Cancer.* 1988;61:989–996.

Norris HJ, Taylor HB. Prognosis of mucinous (gelatinous) carcinoma of the breast. *Cancer.* 1965;18:879–885.

Ranade A, Batra R, Sandhu G, et al. Clinicopathological evaluation of 100 cases of mucinous carcinoma of breast with emphasis on axillary staging and special reference to a micropapillary pattern. *J Clin Pathol.* 2010;63:1043–1047.

Rasmussen BB, Rose C, Christensen IB. Prognostic factors in primary mucinous breast carcinoma. *Am J Clin Pathol.* 1987;87:155–160.

Scopsi L, Andreola S, Pilotti S, et al. Mucinous carcinoma of the breast. A clinicopathologic, histochemical, and immunocytochemical study with special reference to neuroendocrine differentiation. *Am J Surg Pathol.* 1994;18:702–711.

Tan PH, Tse GM, Bay BH. Mucinous breast lesions: diagnostic challenges. *J Clin Pathol.* 2008;61:11–19.

Toikkanen S, Kujari H. Pure and mixed mucinous carcinomas of the breast: a clinicopathologic analysis of 61 cases with long-term follow-up. *Hum Pathol.* 1989;20:758–764.

Weigelt B, Geyer FC, Horlings HM, et al. Mucinous and neuroendocrine breast carcinomas are transcriptionally distinct from invasive ductal carcinomas of no special type. *Mod Pathol.* 2009;22:1401–1414.

Wilson TE, Helvie MA, Oberman HA, et al. Pure and mixed mucinous carcinoma of the breast: pathologic basis for differences in mammographic appearance. *AJR Am J Roentgenol.* 1995;165:285–289.

MEDULLARY CARCINOMA

Dadmanesh F, Peterse JL, Sapino A, et al. Lymphoepithelioma-like carcinoma of the breast: lack of evidence of Epstein-Barr virus infection. *Histopathology.* 2001;38:54–61.

Jacquemier J, Padovani L, Rabayrol L, et al. Typical medullary breast carcinomas have a basal/myoepithelial phenotype. *J Pathol.* 2005;207:260–268.

Kulka J, Kovalszky I, Svastics E, et al. Lymphoepithelioma-like carcinoma of the breast: not Epstein-Barr virus-, but human papilloma virus-positive. *Hum Pathol.* 2008;39:298–301.

Kumar S, Kumar D. Lymphoepithelioma-like carcinoma of the breast. *Mod Pathol.* 1994;7:129–131.

Lakhani SR, Reis-Filho JS, Fulford L, et al. Prediction of BRCA1 status in patients with breast cancer using estrogen receptor and basal phenotype. *Clin Cancer Res.* 2005;11:5175–5180.

Meyer JE, Amin E, Lindfors KK, et al. Medullary carcinoma of the breast: mammographic and US appearance. *Radiology.* 1989;170:79–82.

Rakha EA, Aleskandarany M, El-Sayed ME, et al. The prognostic significance of inflammation and medullary histological type in invasive carcinoma of the breast. *Eur J Cancer.* 2009;45:1780–1787.

Rapin V, Contesso G, Mouriesse H, et al. Medullary breast carcinoma. A reevaluation of 95 cases of breast cancer with inflammatory stroma. *Cancer.* 1988;61:2503–2510.

Ridolfi RL, Rosen PP, Port A, et al. Medullary carcinoma of the breast: a clinicopathologic study with 10 year follow-up. *Cancer.* 1977;40:1365–1385.

Vincent-Salomon A, Gruel N, Lucchesi C, et al. Identification of typical medullary breast carcinoma as a genomic sub-group of basal-like carcinomas, a heterogeneous new molecular entity. *Breast Cancer Res.* 2007;9:R24.

Wargotz ES, Silverberg SG. Medullary carcinoma of the breast: a clinicopathologic study with appraisal of current diagnostic criteria. *Hum Pathol.* 1988;19:1340–1346.

METAPLASTIC CARCINOMA

Al-Bozom IA, Abrams J. Spindle cell carcinoma of the breast, a mimicker of benign lesions: case report and review of the literature. *Arch Pathol Lab Med.* 1996;120:1066–1068.

An T, Grathwohl M, Frable WJ. Breast carcinoma with osseous metaplasia: an electron microscopic study. *Am J Clin Pathol.* 1984;81:127–132.

Barnes PJ, Boutilier R, Chiasson D, et al. Metaplastic breast carcinoma: clinical-pathologic characteristics and HER2/neu expression. *Breast Cancer Res Treat.* 2005;91:173–178.

Chhieng C, Cranor M, Lesser ME, et al. Metaplastic carcinoma of the breast with osteocartilaginous heterologous elements. *Am J Surg Pathol.* 1998;22:188–194.

Cornog JL, Mobini J, Steiger E, et al. Squamous carcinoma of the breast. *Am J Clin Pathol.* 1971;55:410–417.

Downs-Kelly E, Nayeemuddin KM, Albarracin C, et al. Matrix-producing carcinoma of the breast: an aggressive subtype of metaplastic carcinoma. *Am J Surg Pathol.* 2009;33:534–541.

Falconieri G, Della Libera D, Zanconati F, et al. Leiomyosarcoma of the female breast: report of two new cases and a review of the literature. *Am J Clin Pathol.* 1997;108:19–25.

Gobbi H, Simpson JF, Borowsky A, et al. Metaplastic breast tumors with a dominant fibromatosis-like phenotype have a high risk of local recurrence. *Cancer.* 1999;85:2170–2182.

Koker MM, Kleer CG. p63 expression in breast cancer: a highly sensitive and specific marker of metaplastic carcinoma. *Am J Surg Pathol.* 2004;28:1506–1512.

Livasy CA, Karaca G, Nanda R, et al. Phenotypic evaluation of the basal-like subtype of invasive breast carcinoma. *Mod Pathol.* 2006;19:264–271.

Okada N, Hasebe T, Iwasaki M, et al. Metaplastic carcinoma of the breast. *Hum Pathol.* 2010;41:960–970.

Pitts WC, Rojas VA, Gaffey MJ, et al. Carcinomas with metaplasia and sarcomas of the breast. *Am J Clin Pathol.* 1991;95:623–632.

Podetta M, D'Ambrosio G, Ferrari A, et al. Low-grade fibromatosis-like spindle cell metaplastic carcinoma: a basal-like tumor with a favorable clinical outcome. Report of two cases. *Tumori.* 2009;95:264–267.

Sneige N, Yaziji H, Mandavilli SR, et al. Low-grade (fibromatosis-like) spindle cell carcinoma of the breast. *Am J Surg Pathol.* 2001;25:1009–1016.

Tse GM, Tan PH, Chaiwun B, et al. p63 is useful in the diagnosis of mammary metaplastic carcinomas. *Pathology.* 2006;38:16–20.

Tse GM, Tan PH, Putti TC, et al. Metaplastic carcinoma of the breast: a clinicopathological review. *J Clin Pathol.* 2006;59:1079–1083.

Wargotz ES, Deos PH, Norris HJ. Metaplastic carcinomas of the breast. II. Spindle cell carcinoma. *Hum Pathol.* 1989;20:732–740.

Wargotz ES, Norris HJ. Metaplastic carcinomas of the breast. I. Matrix-producing carcinoma. *Hum Pathol.* 1989;20:628–635.

ADENOID CYSTIC CARCINOMA

Crisi GM, Marconi SA, Makari-Judson G, et al. Expression of c-kit in adenoid cystic carcinoma of the breast. *Am J Clin Pathol.* 2005;124:733–739.

Fukuoka K, Hirokawa M, Shimizu M, et al. Basaloid type adenoid cystic carcinoma of the breast. *APMIS.* 1999;107:762–766.

Hodgson NC, Lytwyn A, Bacopulos S, et al. Adenoid cystic breast carcinoma: high rates of margin positivity after breast conserving surgery. *Am J Clin Oncol.* 2010;33:28–31.

Jan YJ, Li MC, Ho WL. Collagenous spherulosis presenting as a mass of the breast. *Zhonghua Yi Xue Za Zhi (Taipei).* 2002;65:494–497.

Kontos M, Fentiman IS. Adenoid cystic carcinoma of the breast. *Int J Clin Pract.* 2003;57:669–672.

Lamovec J, Us-Krasovec M, Zidar A, et al. Adenoid cystic carcinoma of the breast: a histologic, cytologic, and immunohistochemical study. *Semin Diagn Pathol.* 1989;6:153–164.

Marchio C, Weigelt B, Reis-Filho JS. Adenoid cystic carcinomas of the breast and salivary glands (or 'The strange case of Dr Jekyll and Mr Hyde' of exocrine gland carcinomas). *J Clin Pathol.* 2010;63:220–228.

Mastropasqua MG, Maiorano E, Pruneri G, et al. Immunoreactivity for c-kit and p63 as an adjunct in the diagnosis of adenoid cystic carcinoma of the breast. *Mod Pathol.* 2005;18:1277–1282.

Michal M, Skalova A. Collagenous spherulosis. A comment on its histogenesis. *Pathol Res Pract.* 1990;186:365–370.

Pesutic-Pisac V, Bezic J, Tomic S. Collagenous spherulosis of the breast in association with in situ carcinoma. *Pathologica.* 2002;94:317–319.

Ro JY, Silva EG, Gallager HS. Adenoid cystic carcinoma of the breast. *Hum Pathol.* 1987;18:1276–1281.

Sheen-Chen SM, Eng HL, Chen WJ, et al. Adenoid cystic carcinoma of the breast: truly uncommon or easily overlooked? *Anticancer Res.* 2005;25:455–458.

Shin SJ, Rosen PP. Solid variant of mammary adenoid cystic carcinoma with basaloid features: a study of nine cases. *Am J Surg Pathol.* 2002;26:413–420.

Torrao MM, da Costa JM, Ferreira E, et al. Adenoid cystic carcinoma of the breast. *Breast J.* 2007;13:206.

PAPILLARY CARCINOMA

Dogan BE, Whitman GJ, Middleton LP, et al. Intracystic papillary carcinoma of the breast. *AJR Am J Roentgenol.* 2003;181:186.

Fisher ER, Palekar AS, Redmond C, et al. Pathologic findings from the National Surgical Adjuvant Breast Project (protocol no. 4). VI. Invasive papillary cancer. *Am J Clin Pathol.* 1980;73:313–322.

Hall FM. Papillary lesions of the breast. *Radiology.* 2007;243:300–301; author reply 1.

Hill CB, Yeh IT. Myoepithelial cell staining patterns of papillary breast lesions: from intraductal papillomas to invasive papillary carcinomas. *Am J Clin Pathol.* 2005;123:36–44.

Ibarra JA. Papillary lesions of the breast. *Breast J.* 2006;12:237–251.

Koerner F. Papilloma and papillary carcinoma. *Semin Diagn Pathol.* 2010;27:13–30.

Murad TM, Swaid S, Pritchett P. Malignant and benign papillary lesions of the breast. *Hum Pathol.* 1977;8:379–390.

Rabban JT, Koerner FC, Lerwill MF. Solid papillary ductal carcinoma in situ versus usual ductal hyperplasia in the breast: a potentially difficult distinction resolved by cytokeratin 5/6. *Hum Pathol.* 2006;37:787–793.

Raju UB, Lee MW, Zarbo RJ, et al. Papillary neoplasia of the breast: immunohistochemically defined myoepithelial cells in the diagnosis of benign and malignant papillary breast neoplasms. *Mod Pathol.* 1989;2:569–576.

Rosen PP, Hoda SA, Dershaw DD, et al. *Breast Pathology: Diagnosis by Needle Core Biopsy.* 2nd ed. Philadelphia, PA: Lippincott Williams & Wilkins; 2006.

Soo MS, Williford ME, Walsh R, et al. Papillary carcinoma of the breast: imaging findings. *AJR Am J Roentgenol.* 1995;164:321–326.

Stefanou D, Batistatou A, Nonni A, et al. p63 expression in benign and malignant breast lesions. *Histol Histopathol.* 2004;19:465–471.

Wilkes AN, Feig SA, Palazzo JP. Breast imaging case of the day. Intracystic papillary carcinoma of the breast. *Radiographics.* 1998;18:1310–1313.

Wynveen CA, Nehhozina T, Akram M, et al. Intracystic papillary carcinoma of the breast: An in situ or invasive tumor? Results of immunohistochemical analysis and clinical follow-up. *Am J Surg Pathol.* 2011;35:1–14.

4. PROLIFERATIVE STROMAL AND MISCELLANEOUS MESENCHYMAL LESIONS

FIBROADENOMA

Abe M, Miyata S, Nishimura S, et al. Malignant transformation of breast fibroadenoma to malignant phyllodes tumor: long-term outcome of 36 malignant phyllodes tumors. *Breast Cancer.* 2009; Dec 26 2009 epub.

Azzopardi JG, Ahmed A, Millis RR. Problems in breast pathology. *Major Probl Pathol.* 1979;11:i–xvi, 1–466.

Buzanowski-Konakry K, Harrison EG Jr, Payne WS. Lobular carcinoma arising in fibroadenoma of the breast. *Cancer.* 1975;35:450–456.

Carter D. *Interpretation of Breast Biopsies.* 4th ed. Philadelphia, PA: Lippincott Williams & Wilkins; 2003.

Diaz NM, Palmer JO, McDivitt RW. Carcinoma arising within fibroadenomas of the breast. A clinico-pathologic study of 105 patients. *Am J Clin Pathol.* 1991;95:614–622.

Dupont WD, Page DL, Parl FF, et al. Long-term risk of breast cancer in women with fibroadenoma. *N Engl J Med.* 1994;331:10–15.

Ferreira M, Albarracin CT, Resetkova E. Pseudoangiomatous stromal hyperplasia tumor: a clinical, radiologic and pathologic study of 26 cases. *Mod Pathol.* 2008;21:201–207.

Fondo EY, Rosen PP, Fracchia AA, et al. The problem of carcinoma developing in a fibroadenoma: recent experience at Memorial Hospital. *Cancer.* 1979;43:563–567.

Jacobs TW, Chen YY, Guinee DG Jr, et al. Fibroepithelial lesions with cellular stroma on breast core needle biopsy: are there predictors of outcome on surgical excision? *Am J Clin Pathol.* 2005;124:342–354.

Kuijper A, Buerger H, Simon R, et al. Analysis of the progression of fibroepithelial tumours of the breast by PCR-based clonality assay. *J Pathol.* 2002;197:575–581.

Lee AH, Hodi Z, Ellis IO, et al. Histological features useful in the distinction of phyllodes tumour and fibroadenoma on needle core biopsy of the breast. *Histopathology.* 2007;51:336–344.

Mies C, Rosen PP. Juvenile fibroadenoma with atypical epithelial hyperplasia. *Am J Surg Pathol.* 1987;11:184–190.

Moore T, Lee AH. Expression of CD34 and bcl-2 in phyllodes tumours, fibroadenomas and spindle cell lesions of the breast. *Histopathology.* 2001;38:62–67.

Pike AM, Oberman HA. Juvenile (cellular) adenofibromas. A clinicopathologic study. *Am J Surg Pathol.* 1985;9:730–736.

Powell CM, Cranor ML, Rosen PP. Pseudoangiomatous stromal hyperplasia (PASH). A mammary stromal tumor with myofibroblastic differentiation. *Am J Surg Pathol.* 1995;19:270–277.

Tavassoli FA, Eusebi V, American Registry of Pathology, et al. *Tumors of the Mammary Gland.* Washington, D.C.: American Registry of Pathology in collaboration with the Armed Forces Institute of Pathology; 2009.

Vazmitel M, Pavlovsky M, Kacerovska D, et al. Pseudoangiomatous stromal hyperplasia in a complex neoplastic lesion involving anogenital mammary-like glands. *J Cutan Pathol.* 2009;36:1117–1120.

PHYLLODES TUMOR

Azzopardi JG, Ahmed A, Millis RR. Problems in breast pathology. *Major Probl Pathol.* 1979;11:i–xvi, 1–466.

Barth RJ Jr. Histologic features predict local recurrence after breast conserving therapy of phyllodes tumors. *Breast Cancer Res Treat.* 1999;57:291–295.

Carter BA, Page DL. Phyllodes tumor of the breast: local recurrence versus metastatic capacity. *Hum Pathol.* 2004;35:1051–1052.

Chaney AW, Pollack A, McNeese MD, et al. Primary treatment of cystosarcoma phyllodes of the breast. *Cancer.* 2000;89:1502–1511.

Cohn-Cedermark G, Rutqvist L, Rosendahl I, et al. Prognostic factors in cystosarcoma phyllodes. A clinicopathologic study of 77 patients. *Cancer.* 1991;68:2017–2022.

de Roos WK, Kaye P, Dent DM. Factors leading to local recurrence or death after surgical resection of phyllodes tumours of the breast. *Br J Surg.* 1999;86:396–399.

Eroglu E, Irkkan C, Ozsoy M, et al. Phyllodes tumor of the breast: case series of 40 patients. *Eur J Gynaecol Onco.* 2004;25:123–125.

Hart W, Bauer R, HA O. Cystosarcoma phyllodes. A clinicopathologic study of twenty-six hypercellular periductal stromal tumors of the breast. *Am J Clin Pathol.* 1978;70:211–216.

Hawkins RE, Schofield JB, Fisher C, et al. The clinical and histologic criteria that predict metastases from cystosarcoma phyllodes. *Cancer.* 1992;69:141–147.

Jacobs TW, Chen YY, Guinee DG Jr, et al. Fibroepithelial lesions with cellular stroma on breast core needle biopsy: are there predictors of outcome on surgical excision? *Am J Clin Pathol.* 2005;124:342–354.

Jimenez JF, Gloster ES, Perrot LJ, et al. Liposarcoma arising within a cystosarcoma phyllodes. *J Surg Oncol.* 1986;31:294–298.

Kasami M, Vnencak-Jones CL, Manning S, et al. Monoclonality in fibroadenomas with complex histology and phyllodal features. *Breast Cancer Res Treat.* 1998;50:185–191.

Katsohis C, Fahandides E, Agurigakis C, et al. Cystosarcoma phyllodes of the breast. *Int Surg.* 1990;75:162–165.

Keelan P, Myers J, Wold L, et al. Phyllodes tumor: clinicopathologic review of 60 patients and flow cytometric analysis in 30 patients. *Hum Pathol.* 1992;23:1048–1054.

Kuijper A, Buerger H, Simon R, et al. Analysis of the progression of fibroepithelial tumours of the breast by PCR-based clonality assay. *J Pathol.* 2002;197:575–581.

Moffat CJ, Pinder SE, Dixon AR, et al. Phyllodes tumours of the breast: a clinicopathological review of thirty-two cases. *Histopathology*. 1995;27:205-218.

Moore T, Lee AH. Expression of CD34 and bcl-2 in phyllodes tumours, fibroadenomas and spindle cell lesions of the breast. *Histopathology*. 2001;38:62-67.

Noguchi S, Aihara T, Koyama H, et al. Clonal analysis of benign and malignant human breast tumors by means of polymerase chain reaction. *Cancer Lett*. 1995;90:57-63.

Noguchi S, Yokouchi H, Aihara T, et al. Progression of fibroadenoma to phyllodes tumor demonstrated by clonal analysis. *Cancer*. 1995;76:1779-1785.

Powell C, Rosen P. Adipose differentiation in cystosarcoma phyllodes. A study of 14 cases. *Am J Surg Pathol*. 1994;18:720-727.

Qizilbash AH. Cystosarcoma phyllodes with liposarcomatous stroma. *Am J Clin Pathol*. 1976;65:321-327.

Tavassoli FA, Devilee P, International Agency for Research on Cancer, et al. *Pathology and Genetics of Tumours of the Breast and Female Genital Organs*. Lyon, Fracnce: IARC Press; 2003.

Tavassoli FA, Eusebi V, American Registry of Pathology, et al. *Tumors of the Mammary Gland*. Washington, D.C.: American Registry of Pathology in collaboration with the Armed Forces Institute of Pathology; 2009.

Ward RM, Evans HL. Cystosarcoma phyllodes. A clinicopathologic study of 26 cases. *Cancer*. 1986;58:2282-2289.

PERIDUCTAL STROMAL TUMOR

Burga AM, Tavassoli FA. Periductal stromal tumor: a rare lesion with low-grade sarcomatous behavior. *Am J Surg Pathol*. 2003;27:343-348.

Rao AC, Geetha V, Khurana A. Periductal stromal sarcoma of breast with lipoblast-like cells: a case report with review of literature. *Indian J Pathol Microbiol*. 2008;51:252-254.

Tavassoli FA, Devilee P, International Agency for Research on Cancer, et al. *Pathology and Genetics of Tumours of the Breast and Female Genital Organs*. Lyon, France: IARC Press; 2003.

Tavassoli FA, Eusebi V, American Registry of Pathology, et al. *Tumors of the Mammary Gland*. Washington, D.C.: American Registry of Pathology in collaboration with the Armed Forces Institute of Pathology; 2009.

Tomas D, Jankovic D, Marusic Z, et al. Low-grade periductal stromal sarcoma of the breast with myxoid features: immunohistochemistry. *Pathol Int*. 2009;59:588-591.

MYOFIBROBLASTOMA

Damiani S, Miettinen M, Peterse JL, et al. Solitary fibrous tumour (myofibroblastoma) of the breast. *Virchows Arch*. 1994;425:89-92.

Falconieri G, Lamovec J, Mirra M, et al. Solitary fibrous tumor of the mammary gland: a potential pitfall in breast pathology. *Ann Diagn Pathol*. 2004;8:121-125.

Lacroix-Triki M, Geyer FC, Lambros MB, et al. beta-catenin/Wnt signalling pathway in fibromatosis, metaplastic carcinomas and phyllodes tumours of the breast. *Mod Pathol*. 2010;23:1438-1448.

Magro G. Epithelioid-cell myofibroblastoma of the breast: expanding the morphologic spectrum. *Am J Surg Pathol*. 2009;33:1085-1092.

Magro G, Bisceglia M, Michal M, et al. Spindle cell lipoma-like tumor, solitary fibrous tumor and myofibroblastoma of the breast: a clinico-pathological analysis of 13 cases in favor of a unifying histogenetic concept. *Virchows Arch*. 2002;440:249-260.

Magro G, Michal M, Bisceglia M. Benign spindle cell tumors of the mammary stroma: diagnostic criteria, classification, and histogenesis. *Pathol Res Pract*. 2001;197:453-466.

Morgan MB, Pitha JV. Myofibroblastoma of the breast revisited: an etiologic association with androgens? *Hum Pathol*. 1998;29:347-351.

Pauwels P, Sciot R, Croiset F, et al. Myofibroblastoma of the breast: genetic link with spindle cell lipoma. *J Pathol*. 2000;191:282-285.

Powell CM, Cranor ML, Rosen PP. Pseudoangiomatous stromal hyperplasia (PASH). A mammary stromal tumor with myofibroblastic differentiation. *Am J Surg Pathol*. 1995;19:270-277.

Reis-Filho JS, Faoro LN, Gasparetto EL, et al. Mammary epithelioid myofibroblastoma arising in bilateral gynecomastia: case report with immunohistochemical profile. *Int J Surg Pathol.* 2001;9:331–334.

Tavassoli FA, Eusebi V, American Registry of Pathology, et al. *Tumors of the Mammary Gland.* Washington, D.C.: American Registry of Pathology in collaboration with the Armed Forces Institute of Pathology; 2009.

Wahbah MM, Gilcrease MZ, Wu Y. Lipomatous variant of myofibroblastoma with epithelioid features: a rare and diagnostically challenging breast lesion. *Ann Diagn Pathol.* 2010; Oct 28 2010 epub.

Wargotz ES, Weiss SW, Norris HJ. Myofibroblastoma of the breast. Sixteen cases of a distinctive benign mesenchymal tumor. *Am J Surg Pathol.* 1987;11:493–502.

ANGIOSARCOMA

Brenn T, Fletcher CD. Postradiation vascular proliferations: an increasing problem. *Histopathology.* 2006;48:106–114.

Cafiero F, Gipponi M, Peressini A, et al. Radiation-associated angiosarcoma: diagnostic and therapeutic implications–two case reports and a review of the literature. *Cancer.* 1996;77:2496–2502.

Farina MC, Casado V, Renedo G, et al. Epithelioid angiosarcoma of the breast involving the skin: a highly aggressive neoplasm readily mistaken for mammary carcinoma. *J Cutan Pathol.* 2003;30:152–156.

Feigenberg SJ, Mendenhall NP, Reith JD, et al. Angiosarcoma after breast-conserving therapy: experience with hyperfractionated radiotherapy. *Int J Radiat Oncol Biol Phys.* 2002;52:620–626.

Fineberg S, Rosen PP. Cutaneous angiosarcoma and atypical vascular lesions of the skin and breast after radiation therapy for breast carcinoma. *Am J Clin Pathol.* 1994;102:757–763.

Mills TD, Vinnicombe SJ, Wells CA, et al. Angiosarcoma of the breast after wide local excision and radiotherapy for breast carcinoma. *Clin Radiol.* 2002;57:63–66.

Nascimento AF, Raut CP, Fletcher CD. Primary angiosarcoma of the breast: clinicopathologic analysis of 49 cases, suggesting that grade is not prognostic. *Am J Surg Pathol.* 2008;32:1896–1904.

Rosen PP, Kimmel M, Ernsberger D. Mammary angiosarcoma. The prognostic significance of tumor differentiation. *Cancer.* 1988;62:2145–2151.

Scow JS, Reynolds CA, Degnim AC, et al. Primary and secondary angiosarcoma of the breast: the Mayo Clinic experience. *J Surg Oncol.* 2010;101:401–407.

Tavassoli FA, Eusebi V, American Registry of Pathology, et al. *Tumors of the Mammary Gland.* Washington, D.C.: American Registry of Pathology in collaboration with the Armed Forces Institute of Pathology; 2009.

5. METASTATIC TUMORS TO THE BREAST

MELANOMA

Bendic A, Bozic M, Durdov MG. Metaplastic breast carcinoma with melanocytic differentiation. *Pathol Int.* 2009;59:676–680.

Bonetti F, Colombari R, Manfrin E, et al. Breast carcinoma with positive results for melanoma marker (HMB-45). HMB-45 immunoreactivity in normal and neoplastic breast. *Am J Clin Pathol.* 1989;92:491–495.

Di Bonito L, Luchi M, Giarelli L, et al. Metastatic tumors to the female breast. An autopsy study of 12 cases. *Pathol Res Pract.* 1991;187:432–436.

Nobukawa B, Fujii H, Hirai S, et al. Breast carcinoma diverging to aberrant melanocytic differentiation: a case report with histopathologic and loss of heterozygosity analyses. *Am J Surg Pathol.* 1999;23:1280–1287.

Noske A, Schwabe M, Pahl S, et al. Report of a metaplastic carcinoma of the breast with multi-directional differentiation: an adenoid cystic carcinoma, a spindle cell carcinoma and melanoma. *Virchows Arch.* 2008;452:575–579.

Ruffolo EF, Koerner FC, Maluf HM. Metaplastic carcinoma of the breast with melanocytic differentiation. *Mod Pathol.* 1997;10:592–596.

Saitoh K, Saga K, Okazaki M, et al. Pigmented primary carcinoma of the breast: a clinical mimic of malignant melanoma. *Br J Dermatol.* 1998;139:287–290.

MISCELLANEA—OTHER METASTATIC TUMORS

Alexander HR, Turnbull AD, Rosen PP. Isolated breast metastases from gastrointestinal carcinomas: report of two cases. *J Surg Oncol.* 1989;42:264–266.

Balaji R, Ramachandran K, Anila KR. Ovarian carcinoma metastasis to the breast and imaging features with histopathologic correlation: a case report and review of the literature. *Clin Breast Cancer.* 2009;9:196–198.

Dardick L, Comer TP, O'Neill EJ, et al. Metastatic neoplasm presenting as primary cancer of the breast: case reports. *Mil Med.* 1984;149:411–414.

Di Bonito L, Delendi M, Luchi M, et al. Metastases to the breast in patients treated for prostatic carcinoma. *Breast Dis.* 1991;4:141–147.

Di Bonito L, Luchi M, Giarelli L, et al. Metastatic tumors to the female breast. An autopsy study of 12 cases. *Pathol Res Pract.* 1991;187:432–436.

Forte A, Peronace MI, Gallinaro LS, et al. Metastasis to the breast of a renal carcinoma: a clinical case. *Eur Rev Med Pharmacol Sci.* 1999;3:115–118.

Giarelli L, Ferlito A. Bilateral breast metastases from oat-cell lung carcinoma in a man treated with diethylstilbestrol for prostatic adenocarcinoma. *J Am Geriatr Soc.* 1976;24:511–515.

Oshima CT, Wonraht DR, Catarino RM, et al. Estrogen and progesterone receptors in gastric and colorectal cancer. *Hepatogastroenterology.* 1999;46:3155–3158.

Rosen PP, Hoda SA, Dershaw DD, et al. *Breast Pathology: Diagnosis by Needle Core Biopsy.* 2nd ed. Philadelphia, PA: Lippincott Williams & Wilkins; 2006.

Saitoh K, Saga K, Okazaki M, et al. Pigmented primary carcinoma of the breast: a clinical mimic of malignant melanoma. *Br J Dermatol.* 1998;139:287–290.

Tavassoli FA, Eusebi V, American Registry of Pathology, et al. *Tumors of the Mammary Gland.* Washington, D.C.: American Registry of Pathology in collaboration with the Armed Forces Institute of Pathology; 2009.

Wadhwa J, Dawar R, Kumar L. Ovarian carcinoma metastatic to the breast. *Clin Oncol (R Coll Radiol).* 1999;11:419–421.

LYMPHOMA AND HEMATOPOIETIC DISORDERS

Brogi E, Harris NL. Lymphomas of the breast: pathology and clinical behavior. *Semin Oncol.* 1999;26:357–364.

Brooks JJ, Krugman DT, Damjanov I. Myeloid metaplasia presenting as a breast mass. *Am J Surg Pathol.* 1980;4:281–285.

Gholam D, Bibeau F, El Weshi A, et al. Primary breast lymphoma. *Leuk Lymphoma.* 2003;44:1173–1178.

Lamovec J, Jancar J. Primary malignant lymphoma of the breast. Lymphoma of the mucosa-associated lymphoid tissue. *Cancer.* 1987;60:3033–3041.

Mattia AR, Ferry JA, Harris NL. Breast lymphoma. A B-cell spectrum including the low grade B-cell lymphoma of mucosa associated lymphoid tissue. *Am J Surg Pathol.* 1993;17:574–587.

Ribrag V, Bibeau F, El Weshi A, et al. Primary breast lymphoma: a report of 20 cases. *Br J Haematol.* 2001;115:253–256.

Valbuena JR, Admirand JH, Gualco G, et al. Myeloid sarcoma involving the breast. *Arch Pathol Lab Med.* 2005;129:32–38.

Wong WW, Schild SE, Halyard MY, et al. Primary non-Hodgkin lymphoma of the breast: The Mayo Clinic Experience. *J Surg Oncol.* 2002;80:19–25; discussion 6.

Index